AF870833

Malaria - Transmission, Diagnosis and Treatment

Edited by Linda Eva Amoah, Festus Kojo Acquah and Kwame Kumi Asare

Published in London, United Kingdom

Malaria - Transmission, Diagnosis and Treatment
http://dx.doi.org/10.5772/intechopen.107746
Edited by Linda Eva Amoah, Festus Kojo Acquah and Kwame Kumi Asare

Contributors
Apleheni Eunice Melissa Adouko, Arsène Bokulu, Bien-aimé Mandja, Depri Ardiansyah, Deto Ursul Jean-Paul N'guessan, Doudou Batumbo, Emery Metelo, Emile Manzambi, Erick Mukomena, Eulambius Mathias Mlugu, Fiacre Agossa, Fitriani Kahar, Fred Anangwe Amimo, Hyacinthe Lukoki, Ismail Muhammad, Jennifer Afua Afua Afrifa Yamoah, Jonas Bedford Bedford Danquah, Josue Zanga, Mahama Ouattara, Marisol Sandoval-De Mora, Micah Pukuma Sale, Narcisse Basosila, Nurul Qomariyah, S.Y. Didik Widiyanto, Songuigama Coulibaly, Tanko Mahmoud Mohammed, Trésor Iluku, Yuwono Setiadi,

© The Editor(s) and the Author(s) 2024

The rights of the editor(s) and the author(s) have been asserted in accordance with the Copyright, Designs and Patents Act 1988. All rights to the book as a whole are reserved by INTECHOPEN LIMITED. The book as a whole (compilation) cannot be reproduced, distributed or used for commercial or non-commercial purposes without INTECHOPEN LIMITED's written permission. Enquiries concerning the use of the book should be directed to INTECHOPEN LIMITED rights and permissions department (permissions@intechopen.com).
Violations are liable to prosecution under the governing Copyright Law.

Individual chapters of this publication are distributed under the terms of the Creative Commons Attribution 3.0 Unported License which permits commercial use, distribution and reproduction of the individual chapters, provided the original author(s) and source publication are appropriately acknowledged. If so indicated, certain images may not be included under the Creative Commons license. In such cases users will need to obtain permission from the license holder to reproduce the material. More details and guidelines concerning content reuse and adaptation can be found at http://www.intechopen.com/copyright-policy.html.

Notice
Statements and opinions expressed in the chapters are these of the individual contributors and not necessarily those of the editors or publisher. No responsibility is accepted for the accuracy of information contained in the published chapters. The publisher assumes no responsibility for any damage or injury to persons or property arising out of the use of any materials, instructions, methods or ideas contained in the book.

First published in London, United Kingdom, 2024 by IntechOpen
IntechOpen is the global imprint of INTECHOPEN LIMITED, registered in England and Wales, registration number: 11086078, 5 Princes Gate Court, London, SW7 2QJ, United Kingdom
Printed in Croatia

British Library Cataloguing-in-Publication Data
A catalogue record for this book is available from the British Library

Additional hard and PDF copies can be obtained from orders@intechopen.com

Malaria - Transmission, Diagnosis and Treatment
Edited by Linda Eva Amoah, Festus Kojo Acquah and Kwame Kumi Asare
p. cm.

This title is part of the Infectious Diseases Book Series, Volume 29
Topic: Parasitic Infectious Diseases
Series Editor: Alfonso J. Rodriguez-Morales
Topic Editor: Amidou Samie

Print ISBN 978-0-85014-135-1
Online ISBN 978-0-85014-136-8
eBook (PDF) ISBN 978-0-85014-137-5
ISSN 2631-6188

We are IntechOpen, the world's leading publisher of Open Access books

Built by scientists, for scientists

6,900+
Open access books available

185,000+
International authors and editors

200M+
Downloads

156
Countries delivered to

Our authors are among the
Top 1%
most cited scientists

12.2%
Contributors from top 500 universities

CLARIVATE ANALYTICS BOOK CITATION INDEX INDEXED

WEB OF SCIENCE™

Selection of our books indexed in the Book Citation Index
in Web of Science™ Core Collection (BKCI)

Interested in publishing with us?
Contact book.department@intechopen.com

Numbers displayed above are based on latest data collected.
For more information visit www.intechopen.com

IntechOpen Book Series

Infectious Diseases

Volume 29

Aims and Scope of the Series

This series will provide a comprehensive overview of recent research trends in various Infectious Diseases (as per the most recent Baltimore classification). Topics will include general overviews of infections, immunopathology, diagnosis, treatment, epidemiology, etiology, and current clinical recommendations for managing infectious diseases. Ongoing issues, recent advances, and future diagnostic approaches and therapeutic strategies will also be discussed. This book series will focus on various aspects and properties of infectious diseases whose deep understanding is essential for safeguarding the human race from losing resources and economies due to pathogens.

Meet the Series Editor

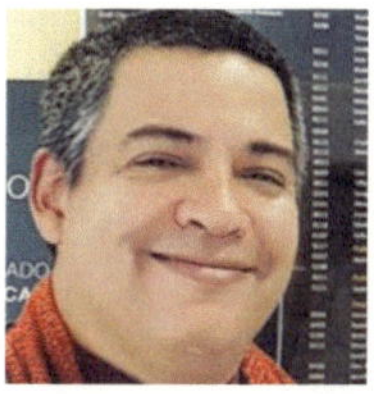

Dr. Rodriguez-Morales is an expert in tropical and emerging diseases, particularly zoonotic and vector-borne diseases (notably arboviral diseases), and more recently COVID-19 and Monkeypox. He is the president of the Publications and Research Committee of the Pan-American Infectious Diseases Association (API), as well as the president of the Colombian Association of Infectious Diseases (ACIN). He is a member of the Committee on Tropical Medicine, Zoonoses, and Travel Medicine of ACIN. Dr. Rodriguez-Morales is a vice-president of the Latin American Society for Travel Medicine (SLAMVI) and a member of the Council of the International Society for Infectious Diseases (ISID). Since 2014, he has been recognized as a senior researcher at the Ministry of Science of Colombia. He is a professor at the Faculty of Medicine of the Fundacion Universitaria Autonoma de las Americas, in Pereira, Risaralda, Colombia, and a professor, Master in Clinical Epidemiology and Biostatistics, at Universidad Científica del Sur, Lima, Peru. He is also a non-resident adjunct faculty member at the Gilbert and Rose-Marie Chagoury School of Medicine, Lebanese American University, Beirut, Lebanon, and an external professor, Master in Research on Tropical Medicine and International Health, at Universitat de Barcelona, Spain. Additionally, an invited professor, Master in Biomedicine, at Universidad Internacional SEK, Quito, Ecuador, and a visiting professor, Master Program of Epidemiology, at Diponegoro University, Indonesia. In 2021 he was awarded the "Raul Isturiz Award" Medal of the API and, the same year, the "Jose Felix Patiño" Asclepius Staff Medal of the Colombian Medical College due to his scientific contributions to the topic of COVID-19 during the pandemic. He is currently the Editor in Chief of the journal Travel Medicine and Infectious Diseases. His Scopus H index is 55 (Google Scholar H index 77) with a total of 725 publications indexed in Scopus.

Meet the Volume Editors

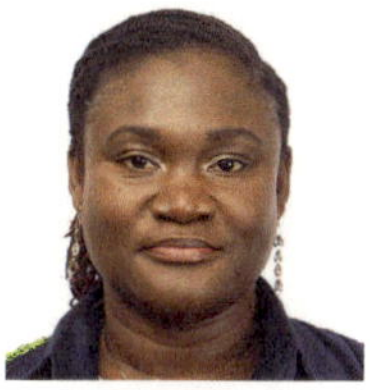

Linda Eva Amoah, Associate Professor of Immunology at the University of Ghana's Noguchi Memorial Institute, specializes in malaria elimination, malaria diagnostics, asymptomatic infections, gametocyte biology, and transmission-blocking immunity. She is the Principal Investigator for several grants, including some awarded by the Bill and Melinda Gates Foundation, National Institutes of Health (NIH), and the Research Institute for Development (IRD). She serves on the editorial board for Frontiers and other journals and has published more than seventy scientific articles.

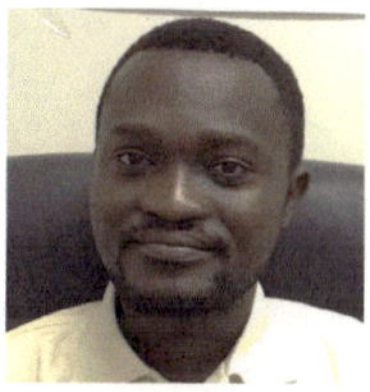

Festus Kojo Acquah, a postdoctoral research fellow at the University of Ghana's Noguchi Memorial Institute for Medical Research, has expertise in protein purification, malaria parasite cultures and drug assays, mosquito standard protocols, and gene cloning. He has published several scientific articles.

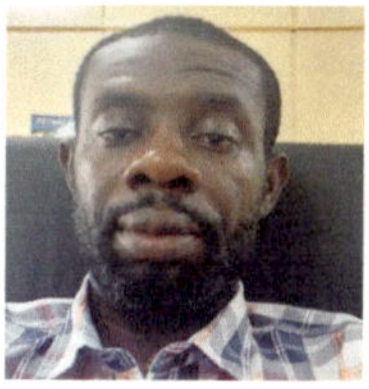

Kwame Kumi Asare, Ph.D., is a biomedical scientist with expertise in infectious and non-communicable diseases and a research fellow at the University of Cape Coast. He has published several scientific articles.

Contents

Preface

Malaria is a major public health issue in sub-Saharan Africa, affecting communities and healthcare systems. Rural communities' knowledge and practices are crucial for malaria prevention and control efforts. Understanding transmission mechanisms, control measures, and modeling is essential for developing effective intervention strategies. Community perceptions and experiences about malaria prevention interventions, such as insecticide-treated bed nets, influence their acceptability and effectiveness. Addressing treatment-seeking behavior, particularly in vulnerable urban populations, is crucial. In-depth qualitative studies are needed to inform targeted interventions. Integrated malaria prevention approaches, including mosquito control, have shown promising results in reducing malaria incidence. However, challenges like low knowledge among migrant farmers and over-treatment in different transmission dynamics need to be addressed. This book provides a contemporary overview of the most important findings in malaria research during the previous few years. The book has four sections.

Section 1 provides an "Overview of Malaria", including information on malaria transmission, diagnosis, treatment, and prevention. It discusses the global public health concern of malaria, malaria prevalence, transmission mechanisms, treatment, control measures, and how modeling is essential for developing effective intervention strategies.

Section 2, "Malaria Transmission", covers perspectives of One Health, zoonotic malaria, environmental transmission, sentinel site and transmission dynamics, and the emergence of insecticide resistance. Malaria transmission is a complex process influenced by environmental, biological, and socioeconomic factors. Topographic features, meteorological conditions, and vector distribution contribute to the disease's transmission. Human activities, such as agricultural practices, can also affect the transmission of malaria. Local-scale hotspots and seasonal migrant workers can resurgence in certain regions. Understanding the spatio-temporal dynamics of malaria is crucial for targeted control strategies. Integrated vector management strategies are effective in controlling transmission, but strategic planning and operational frameworks are needed. Citizen science can monitor vector dynamics and install long-lasting insecticidal nets to break the chain of transmission. Understanding these factors is essential for developing targeted and effective malaria control interventions.

Section 3, "Malaria Diagnosis", discusses the contemporary breakthroughs in malaria diagnosis advancement and the use of unusual sample types. Malaria diagnosis is crucial for disease management, especially in developing countries. Traditional methods like blood examinations are outdated, but newer techniques like antigen tests and polymerase chain reaction (PCR) are gaining traction due to their higher specificity and sensitivity.

Section 4, "Malaria Treatment", focuses on malaria treatment landscapes, current trends, and future perspectives with particular interest in the combination therapy of quinoline nucleus and artemisinin derivatives for the management of uncomplicated malaria. Malaria treatment has evolved, focusing on developing effective drugs. However, drug-resistant *Plasmodium falciparum* strains pose challenges, necessitating individualized drug choices based on disease severity, form, and agent resistance. Widespread resistance hinders antifolates and aminoquinolines in chemotherapy.

This book is required reading for anyone interested in the current state of malaria control efforts, challenges including drug and insecticide resistance, the high cost of control tools, and efforts to develop new tools and genetic control strategies.

Linda Eva Amoah (Ph.D.) and Festus Kojo Acquah (Ph.D.)
Department of Immunology,
Noguchi Memorial Institute for Medical Research,
University of Ghana,
Accra, Ghana

Kwame Kumi Asare (Ph.D.)
Biomedical and Clinical Research Centre,
University of Cape Coast,
Cape Coast, Ghana

Acknowledgement

First and foremost, we want to thank everyone who assisted in the publication of this book. Typists and photographers were among those who worked on this book, as were proofreaders, editors, and content consultants. We want to thank each chapter contributor personally for taking time out of their busy schedules to write the chapters and revise and update information as needed. All these people's efforts, support, and passion were crucial in developing this book for publication. We apologize in advance for those we may have overlooked.

Section 1

Overview of Malaria

Chapter 1

Malaria-Transmission-Diagnosis and Treatment

Marisol Sandoval-De Mora

Abstract

Malaria is a potentially fatal infectious disease, considered a serious public health problem in the world, caused by a parasite of the *Plasmodium* genus. It is transmitted by the bite of the infected female *Anopheles* mosquito, also after blood transfusions, organ transplantation, sharing contaminated syringes in parenteral drug users, in hospitals, and during pregnancy by vertical transmission. The possibility of diagnosis should be considered in any patient with fever during the stay or return from an endemic area, applying microscopy examination through thick drop and smear, rapid diagnostic tests (RDTs), and molecular diagnostic tests (PCR). Specific treatment is based on the parasite species identified, drug resistance, severity of symptoms, or presence of mixed infection. Treatment is based on oral or intravenous artemisinin and severe forms may require supportive measures and surveillance in intensive care units. This chapter aims to provide knowledge about the dynamics of malarial infection, with emphasis on transmission, diagnostic methods, *Plasmodium* species, and current treatment regimen.

Keywords: fever, microscopy, PCR, RDTs, artemisinin, treatment regimen

1. Introduction

Malaria is an infectious disease caused by a *Plasmodium* parasite, which is transmitted by the bite of an infected mosquito, of which the main vector is the female of the genus *Anopheles* [1].

The high number of malaria cases in 2021 (241 million) and deaths (627,000) reveal the fragility of medical services. Especially in the African region where 96% of all deaths were due to malaria, and 80% in children under 5 years of age, more efforts are needed to reverse the trends of recent years. Globally, the number of people at risk of acquiring the disease is high and in areas of high transmission, the most affected with the development of severe disease and death are children and pregnant women. In 2019, it ranked 6th among the leading causes of death in low-resource countries [1–3].

Symptoms of the disease may include the classic form of manifestation "fever, sweating and chills" that appear 10–15 days after the mosquito bite; in addition, headache and vomiting, among others, may be associated. To make the diagnosis, microscopic studies of the patient's blood, such as thick and thin blood smear, are required. Rapid diagnostic tests (RDTs) are also available to identify malaria in dispersed rural areas, with difficult geographical access and without infrastructure for microscopic diagnosis [1, 4].

There are five species of *Plasmodium* responsible for producing the disease in humans, the most frequent being *P. vivax, P. falciparum*, and *P. malariae* and *P. ovale* are rarer. Some primate malarial parasites such as *P. knowlesi, P. cynomolgi, and P. simium* can also infect humans and *P. knowlesi* is mentioned as a species that is naturally transmitted to macaques in Southeast Asia and infects humans causing "zoonotic" malaria; cases have been described in Malaysia with hyperparasitemia and severe complications that can lead to death [4, 5].

Of all these, *P. falciparum* infection is the most severe and causes several clinical conditions of organ damage, called complicated malaria; it can be fatal, if not treated in time [4, 6].

Chloroquine was the drug of choice for malaria and is still administered in most countries to treat *P. vivax* infection; however, it is rarely used in cases of *P. falciparum* because there is currently disseminated resistance to it; therefore, Artemisinin-based combination therapies (ACTs) are now recommended as the main treatment for this parasitic species [1].

In this chapter, the special relevance of this disease in the world will be discussed, with the general objective being to present updated knowledge on general aspects of malaria, its transmission mode, diagnostic methods, and recommended treatment.

2. Transmission

Malaria occurs mainly in tropical regions of sub-Saharan Africa, Asia, Oceania, and Latin America and is transmitted, as previously described, by the bite of the infected female *Anopheles* mosquito. Other forms of transmission are: through blood transfusions, organ transplantation, use of contaminated syringes in intravenous drug users, in hospitals where syringes are reused, and from mother to fetus (called gestational malaria) [4–5].

2.1 High and low transmission areas

Devastating epidemics can occur when the parasite is introduced into an area where the population has had little contact with it and lacks immunity, or when people living in malaria-free areas move to regions where the disease is endemic and can be triggered by climatic conditions, aggravated by natural phenomena such as floods or massive population movements caused by conflicts [1].

The World Health Organization (WHO) recommends the use of different categories depending on the magnitude of transmission according to the situation of each region, the annual parasite incidence, and prevalence of *P. falciparum and P. falciparum/P. vivax* infection [2]:

- High transmission when there is an annual parasite incidence of 450 or more cases per 1000 population and the prevalence of P. *falciparum* malaria is ≥35%.
- Moderate transmission if there is an annual parasite incidence of 250–450 cases per 1000 population and the prevalence of *P. falciparum/ P. vivax* malaria is 10–35%.

- Low transmission if there is an annual incidence of 100–250 cases per 1000 population and the prevalence of *P. falciparum/ P. vivax* malaria is 1–10%.
- Very low transmission areas have an annual parasite incidence of less than 100 cases per 1000 population and the prevalence of *P. falciparum/ P. vivax* malaria is greater than zero but less than 1% [7].

Differences in propagation from one area to another may be due to geographic characteristics, parasite species and vector distribution, socio-demographic characteristics, access to antimalarial treatment, and extensive vector control [8].

A serious problem is the presence of asymptomatic people with malaria and its impact on the transmission and prevalence of the disease, which usually goes unnoticed. They are reservoirs and constitute a focus of infection for people without immunity, which should keep control programs alert in order to initiate and maintain a surveillance system for the early diagnosis of these people, active case detection is important to diagnose these patients. In 2010, in Amazonas state, Venezuela, 81% of PCR tests for *Plasmodium spp.* were diagnosed in asymptomatic persons [9].

3. Diagnosis

Clinical suspicion of malaria is established in any patient with fever during the stay or upon return from an endemic area. Diagnostic tests for this entity are: thick and thin blood smears (gold standard), rapid diagnostic tests (RDTs), and PCR molecular diagnostic tests [4].

Symptoms and signs are nonspecific; suspicion is raised primarily on clinical grounds, based on fever. In endemic areas, any patient with temperature $\geq$ 37.5°C should be considered for confirmation with a parasitological test; results should preferably be available in less than 2 hours.

Parasitological diagnosis: The two methods routinely used to identify microorganisms are: optical microscopy and immunochromatography, the latter detects specific antigens of the parasite or its enzymes that are genus or species specific.

In almost all cases of symptomatic malaria, thick and thin blood smears performed by a competent microscopist will reveal the presence of malarial parasites [2, 4].

3.1 Diagnosis of malaria

In patients with suspected malaria and in other risk groups such as those living with human immunodeficiency virus/acquired immunodeficiency syndrome (HIV/AIDS), the absence of a parasitological diagnosis should not delay the initiation of antimalarial treatment, which should be started immediately.

3.2 Optical microscopy

Microscopic results have not only high sensitivity and specificity for the diagnosis of malaria but also allow quantification of the magnitude of the infection and the parasite species involved. However, the use of this diagnostic resource is costly because it requires the experience and vigilance of the personnel.

Although molecular biology tests are more sensitive, the thick blood smear is still considered the "field standard" against which the sensitivity and specificity of other methods must be compared [10].

Therefore, microscopic examination provides good specificity for the diagnosis of malaria as a febrile illness present. Other important advantages of light microscopy are:

- Low direct costs.
- High sensitivity.
- Differentiation of *Plasmodium* species.
- Determination of the parasite density.
- Detection of gametocytes.
- Follow-up of response to therapy.
- Other infectious agents can be visualized [11].

Numerous tests have been done to improve it, but none have proven superior to the classical Giemsa and immersion oil staining method [2, 12].

3.3 Rapid diagnostic test (RDTs)

There are several tests, which are increasingly useful to complement microscopic findings [13–15].

Rapid diagnostic tests detect by immunochromatography specific *Plasmodium* antigens in the blood of people with malaria. Some tests identify a single species (*P. falciparum*); others identify one or more of the other parasites that affect humans [16–18].

They are commercially available, in strips, cassettes and cards, and easy to use. They are relatively simple to execute and interpret and do not require electricity or special equipment [16, 19].

Since 2012, the World Health Organization (WHO) has recommended that these tests should be selected according to criteria based on contribution results from the WHO Malaria RDT Product Testing program [2, 20].

Current tests are based on the detection of histidine-rich protein 2 (PfHRP2), which is specific for *P. falciparum,* pan-specific or species-specific *Plasmodium* lactate dehydrogenase (LDH), or pan-specific aldolase [2, 21–23].

They have potential advantages including:

- Provides rapid results and extension of diagnostic services to lower levels of health care and communities.
- Few requirements for staff training and skills.
- Strengthening of patient confidence in diagnosis and health service in general.

Disadvantages:

- In countries of the Amazon region, HRP2 deletion in *P. falciparum* exists in variable frequency, making HRP2-based tests not useful in that area [24].
- PfHRP2-based tests cannot distinguish new infections after recent infection, due to the persistence of PfHRP2 in blood for 1–5 weeks after effective therapy [25].
- Poor sensitivity to detect *P. malariae and P. ovale.*
- The heterogeneous quality of commercial products available [2].

3.4 Immunodiagnostic and nucleic acid amplification test methods

Immunodiagnostic tests directly detect the presence of the parasite by capturing parasite antigens during infection, which can be useful for epidemiological studies but lack sensitivity [26].

Techniques to detect nucleic acids such as polymerase chain reaction (PCR) and loop-mediated isothermal amplification are highly sensitive and useful for detecting mixed infection, particularly when there is a low degree of parasitemia, not detectable by light microscopy or with RDTs. They are recommended for drug resistance and epidemiological studies, but their use is not recommended in malaria-endemic areas for routine diagnosis.

So far, nucleic acid amplification tests do not play a role in the clinical management of malaria or in surveillance systems [2, 27].

It is worth noting that malaria surveillance programs should use conventional methods for diagnosis: thick blood smears and RDTs, and leave molecular tests (PCR) for special situations. At the community level, clinical symptoms suggestive of the disease can be used to initiate treatment when RDTs are not available. While in primary care centers, thick blood smears or RDTs or both should be used to decide on treatment. In secondary or tertiary care, light microscopy is important to confirm the diagnosis, measure parasitemia and control follow-up, and only if there are an excessive number of patients, the use of RDTs is preferred. Some patients negative to microscopy and RDTs may have a low degree of parasitemia and will only be diagnosed by performing PCR, which is a more sensitive method [9, 28]

4. Treatment

Treatment depends on the *Plasmodium* species, severity of the disease, drug resistance, age of the patient, and pregnancy [2, 4].

4.1 Treatment of uncomplicated *P. falciparum* malaria

Uncomplicated malaria is defined as a patient who presents symptoms and signs of this entity (fever, myalgia, among others) and a positive parasitological examination (microscopy or RDTs) without features of severity and the objectives of treatment are to cure the infection as quickly as possible and prevent the progression to severe disease [2].

4.2 Artemisinin-based combination therapy (ACTs)

For this clinical form, artemisinin combinations (ACTs) are available, with duration of 3 days and covering two asexual cycles. In relation to the doses, they must be optimal to guarantee rapid clinical and parasitological cure, decrease transmission, and avoid drug resistance [2, 4, 6].

The WHO recommends the following treatment regimens: [2].

4.2.1 Artemether + Lumefantrine

Dosage of 5–24 mg/kg/bw of artemether and 29–144 mg/kg/bw of lumefantrine; administer twice daily, for 3 days (total of 6 doses), the first 2 doses should be given 8 hours apart.

The formulations currently available are tablets of 20 mg of artemether and 120 mg of lumefantrine and another presentation of 40 mg of artemether and 240 mg of lumefantrine, in fixed doses and in combination formulation.

4.2.2 Artesunate + Amodiaquine

Dosage of 4 mg/kg/bw artesunate and 10 mg/kg/bw amodiaquine, once daily for 3 days. A total therapeutic dose of 6–30 mg/kg/bw artesunate and 22.5–45 mg/kg/bw amodiaquine daily dose is recommended.

Available formulations: fixed-dose combination in tablets of 25 + 67.5 mg, 50 + 135 mg, or 100 + 270 mg of artesunate and amodiaquine respectively.

Adverse effects described: severe neutropenia, particularly in patients co-infected with HIV receiving antiretroviral therapy (zidovudine) and/or clotrimoxazole. Concomitant use of efavirenz increases exposure to amodiaquine and the risk of hepatotoxicity. These combinations should be avoided unless it is the only ACTs available.

4.2.3 Artesunate + Mefloquine

Doses of 4 mg/kg/bw per day of artesunate and 8.3 mg/kg/bw per day of mefloquine, once daily for 3 days.

A pediatric tablet formulation of 25 mg artesunate and 5.5 mg mefloquine hydrochloride (equivalent to 50 mg mefloquine base) and adult tablets with 100 mg artesunate and 220 mg mefloquine hydrochloride (equivalent to 200 mg mefloquine base) are available.

Mefloquine is associated with nausea, vomiting, dyskinesia, dysphoria and sleep disturbances, and has been well tolerated. Combination with rifampicin reduces its efficacy.

4.2.4 Artesunate + Sulfadoxine-pyrimethamine

Currently available in 50 mg artesunate tablets and fixed-dose combination tablets with 500 mg sulfadoxine +25 mg pyrimethamine; the dose is 4 mg/kg/bw per day of artesunate for 3 days and a single administration of 25/1.25 mg/kg/bw of sulfadoxine-pyrimethamine, single dose on day 1 of treatment.

4.2.5 Dihydroartemisinin + piperaquine

With the use of this drug the cure rate is excellent (>95%), although in children under 5 years of age, the risk of therapeutic failure is increased by three times. The recommended doses are 4 mg/kg/bw per day of Dihydroartemisinin and 18 mg/kg/bw per day of piperaquine, daily for 3 days for adults and children weighing ≥25 kg. Children weighing less than 25 kg should receive a minimum of 2.5 mg/kg/bw per day of Dihydroartemisinin, and 20 mg/kg/bw per day of piperaquine daily for 3 days. It is available as a fixed-dose combination in tablets of 40 mg Dihydroartemisinin and 320 mg piperaquine and pediatric tablets with 20 mg Dihydroartemisinin and 160 mg piperaquine.

There are factors that alter the efficacy of the drug and the response to therapy: the ingestion of high-fat meals modifies the absorption of piperaquine and increases the risk of arrhythmias, delayed ventricular repolarization with prolongation of the corrected QT interval in the electrocardiogram, and malnourished children are at high risk of not obtaining an adequate response [2, 29, 30].

4.3 Treatment of uncomplicated malaria caused by *P. vivax, P. ovale, P. malariae*, and *P. knowlesi*

The goal of treatment of *P. vivax* malaria is twofold: to cure the acute infection in the blood and to clear the hypnozoites from the liver to prevent relapse.

In areas where *P. vivax* is sensitive to chloroquine, treatment of malaria with oral chloroquine at a dose of 25 mg/kg/bw is effective and well tolerated. It is started with a dose of 10 mg/kg/bw on the first day, continued on the second day with 10 mg/kg/bw and it is ended on the third day with 5 mg/kg/bw.

ACTs are highly effective in the treatment of this parasitic species in areas where chloroquine-resistant *P. vivax* exists; ACTs containing piperaquine, mefloquine, lumefantrine are recommended.

In the therapy of uncomplicated *P. ovale, P. malariae*, and *P. knowlesi* malaria, the resistance of these species to these drugs has not been well characterized, and they are considered sensitive to chloroquine and should be treated with standard chloroquine or ACT regimens [2].

Tafenoquine: It is a new drug belonging to the family of 8-aminoquinoleins. It was discovered in 1978, in response to the search for a drug that acts on acute and latent forms of *P. vivax* infection and although the mechanism of action is not exactly known, it is hypothesized that it induces spontaneous oxidation by redox cycles, causing the death of the parasite. It has few adverse effects, and they occur in approximately 13%, predominantly gastrointestinal symptoms, vortex keratopathy without sequelae, prolongation of the QT interval, and hemolytic anemia in people with G6PD deficiency. In three studies subjected to meta-analysis, the efficacy of treatment with tafenoquine compared to primaquine was evaluated and showed no inferiority, being an alternative that improves treatment compliance and is administered in a single dose [31].

4.4 Mixed malaria

Common in endemic areas, ACTs are effective against all malaria species and are the shock treatment for mixed infections [2].

4.5 Use of primaquine in the treatment of malaria

To reduce the transmissibility of *P. falciparum* infection in areas of low transmission intensity, it should be administered in a single dose of 0.25 mg/kg/bw and accompanied by ACTs (except in pregnant women, children under 6 months of age, and women breastfeeding children under 6 months of age).

To prevent relapses in *P. vivax* malaria, *P. ovale* in children and adults (except pregnant women, children under 6 months, women breastfeeding children under 6 months, and persons with G6PD deficiency) should be treated with primaquine at doses of 0.25–0.50 mg/kg/bw, once daily for 14 days [2, 4].

4.6 Treatment of severe malaria

Treatment includes a general approach and the use of antimalarial drugs; general measures include: parenteral hydration, transfusion of globular or platelet concentrates; according to the patient's condition. In situations of advanced clinical deterioration, nutritional support, renal replacement therapy (hemodialysis), and mechanical ventilation may be required.

Severe malaria is a medical emergency, and it is essential to perform supportive measures and give full and effective parenteral or rectal doses of antimalarial drugs in the initial treatment. Two groups of drugs are available for intravenous administration: artemisinin derivatives (artesunate or artemether) and cinchona alkaloids (quinine and quinidine) [2, 4, 6, 32, 33].

The clinical and rapid assessment with emphasis on the patient's general condition includes: assessing the state of consciousness using the Glasgow scale, quantifying vital signs (blood pressure, frequency, and depth of respiration), as well as the degree of skin pallor.

General treatment for severe malaria and its complications:

1. Immediately hospitalize.

2. Close and continuous monitoring of vital signs and hemodynamic parameters.

3. Maintain general metabolic functions.

4. Immediate indication of specific antimalarial chemotherapy.

5. Medical work in a multidisciplinary team: internists, pediatricians, infectious disease specialists, obstetrician-gynecologists, intensivists, nephrologists, hematologists, epidemiologists.

6. Admission to the intensive care unit (ICU) or intermediate care unit for close monitoring.

7. To ensure airway patency, place cannula.

8. If hypoxia (oxygen saturation < 90%) administer oxygen.

9. In respiratory failure, manual or oxygen-assisted ventilation can be initiated.

10. Place bladder catheter for control of liquids eliminated, record the water balance including inflow and outflow.

11. Process priority and immediate tests such as thick and thin blood smear and rapid diagnostic tests (RDTs), complete hematology, glycemia, serum electrolytes, total and fractionated bilirubin, transaminases, urea, and creatinine.

12. Perform peripheral blood smears every 12 hours to determine parasitemia during the first 2–3 days.

13. Administer paracetamol or acetaminophen. Do not give NSAIDs or steroids.

Hydration: If there is no evidence of fluid overload, patients with oral intolerance (adults and pediatric) should receive 5% dextrose solutions, and those who tolerate the oral route, administer isotonic saline solution at a rate of 1–2 mL/kg/hour. Take care not to overhydrate the patient [2, 6].

Treatment of anemia: In adults, if the hematocrit <20 or Hb < 7 g/dL, transfuse whole blood or packed red cells over 6 hours [2, 6].

The advantages of artemisinin over quinine are evident, demonstrating a decrease in mortality with the administration of artesunate; it is simple and safe, it is applied in bolus intravenously or intramuscularly, without the adverse effects of quinine, nor the difficulties of intravenous dilution several times a day [2, 6, 32–34].

Antimalarial drugs: In any case of severe malaria, antimalarial chemotherapy should be initiated early [2, 4, 6, 35–40].

First line in severe malaria: The therapeutic scheme is of international use.

Artesunate: WHO (2012) has indicated that the isolated use of this parenteral drug is the initial treatment of choice for this clinical form, the benefit is due to the fact that rapid therapeutic plasma concentrations are obtained, it is well tolerated, unlike quinine it eliminates parasitemia faster and has few adverse effects, it can be administered intravenously or intramuscularly [40].

Dosage according to patient's weight:

a. Patient with less than 20 kg: 3 mg/kg/bw/dose.

b. Patient ≥20 kg: 2.4 mg/kg/bw/dose.

The first three doses of Artesunate are administered following an hourly interval; the first, upon admission (hour 0); the second 12 hours after the previous one and the third, 24 hours after the initial dose; with the option of prescribing additional doses, if the patient requires it. In this situation, continue with the medication until oral tolerance is recovered and a maximum of 7 days. Once the oral route is recovered, full therapy with Artemether 20 mg + Lumefantrine 120 mg for 3 days plus Primaquine at 0.50 mg/kg bw in a single dose is prescribed in case of *P. falciparum infection,* or in case of *P. vivax* or mixed infections at 0.25 mg/kg bw daily for 14 days.

Artemether attack dose: 3.2 mg/kg/bw and maintenance dose: 1.6 mg/kg/bw. First dose at admission (hour 0), then a maintenance dose every 24 hours until oral tolerance is achieved, for a maximum of 5 days. When tolerance is restored, oral treatment with Artemether 20 mg + Lumefantrine 120 mg for 3 days plus Primaquine at 0.50 mg/kg bw in a single dose in case of *P. falciparum infection*, or 0.25 mg/kg bw, daily for 14 days in case of *P. vivax* or mixed infections.

Quinine dihydrochloride dose of 10 mgs/kg/bw + Clindamycin 10 mgs/kg/bw, both intravenously. First dose at admission (hour 0), continue with Quinine every 8 hours plus Clindamycin every 12 hours until oral tolerance is recovered, for a maximum of 7 days. Depending on oral availability, complete 7 days with Quinine in tablets at 10 mg/kg bw every 8 hours, plus Clindamycin at 10 mg/kg bw every 12 hours for 7 days or Doxycycline at 4 mg/kg bw per day for 7 days, plus Primaquine at 0.50 mg/kg bw in single dose in case of *P. falciparum infection*, or 0.25 mg/kg bw per day for 14 days in case of *P. vivax* or mixed infection [2, 4, 34, 36–41].

Some authors propose giving high, supervised doses of Primaquine at 7 mgs/kg/bw day for 14 days to reduce relapses of *P. vivax* and *P. falciparum* malaria [42–43].

5. Conclusions

In this chapter, the review of national and international literature related to malaria shows its importance worldwide as a potentially fatal disease, is transmissible in tropical countries, more frequent in Africa, Asia, Oceania, and Latin America; the alternative diagnostic methods are exposed with their strengths and weaknesses, especially the parasitological ones with the thick blood smear as the gold standard, accompanied by thin blood smear; also, the usefulness of RDTs in remote sites, where microscopy is not available for an immediate diagnosis. In relation to antimalarial treatment, the current guidelines and recommendations are presented with the use of Artemisinin combinations (ACTs) and their different presentations for the therapy of uncomplicated *P. falciparum* malaria, or in mixed malaria, and the conduct in case of severe malaria with the use of ACTs in their different forms of administration: oral, rectal, intramuscular, and intravenous. Finally, the indication of primaquine and tafenoquine to avoid relapses and contagion of this entity; without diagnostic delay and early initiation of medication to prevent fatal outcomes due to severe complications, we should be waiting for updates on the different diagnostic, therapeutic, and preventive options, as long as the fight toward the eradication of this disease is a reality in the world.

Acknowledgements

The author acknowledges to Dr. María Eugenia Guzmán Siritt, for her contributions to the review of the chapter.

Conflict of interest

"The author declares no conflict of interest".

DOI: http://dx.doi.org/10.5772/intechopen.113746

Author details

Marisol Sandoval-De Mora
Universidad de Oriente, School of Health Sciences "Dr Francisco Battistini Casalta", Ciudad Bolívar, Venezuela

*Address all correspondence to: sandomarisol@gmail.com

IntechOpen

© 2023 The Author(s). Licensee IntechOpen. This chapter is distributed under the terms of the Creative Commons Attribution License (http://creativecommons.org/licenses/by/3.0), which permits unrestricted use, distribution, and reproduction in any medium, provided the original work is properly cited.

References

[1] Pan American Health Organization (PAHO) and World Health Organization (WHO). Malaria [Online]. 2020. Available from: https://www.paho.org.int [Accessed: 07 July, 2023]

[2] World Health Organization (2023). WHO guidelines on malaria. World Health Organization. License: CC BY-NC-SA 3.0 IGO. 14 March 2023. Available from: https://apps.who.int/iris/handle/10665/366432 [Accessed: 07 June 2023]

[3] World Malaria Report 2022. Geneva: World Health Organization. License: CC BY-NC-SA 3.0 IGO. 2022. Available from: https://www.who.int/teams/global-malaria-programme/reports/world-malaria-report-2022 [Accessed: 20 July 2023]

[4] Fairhurst R, Wellems T. Malaria (*Plasmodium* species). In: Bennett JE, Dolin R, Blaser MJ, Mandell GL, Douglas RG, editors. Principles and Practice of Infectious Diseases. 9th ed. Philadelphia, PA: Elseiver/Saunders; 2020. pp. 3299-3320

[5] Mace KE, Arguin PM, Tan KR. Malaria surveillance-United States, 2015. MMWR Surveillance Summary. 2018;**67**(SS-7):1-28. DOI: 10.15585/mmwr.ss6707a1 [Accessed: 14 July 2023]

[6] Sandoval de Mora M. Clinical and therapeutic management of severe malaria. Boletin Venez Infectol. 2022;**33**(1):24-29. DOI: 10.54868/BVI.2022.33.1.3

[7] Yekutiel P. Problems of epidemiology in malaria eradication. Bulletin of the World Health Organization. 1960;**22**(6):669-683. Available from: https://apps.who.int/iris/handle/10665/267282 [Accessed: July 14, 2023]

[8] Cameron E, Battle KE, Bhatt S, Weiss DJ, Bisanzio D, Mappin B, et al. Defining the relationship between prevalence of infection and clinical incidence of plasmodium falciparum malaria. Nature Communications. 2015;**6**:8170. DOI: 10.1038/ncomms9170

[9] Rodríguez I, De Abreu N, Carrasquel A, Bolívar J, González M, Scorza JV, et al. Malarial infections in asymptomatic individuals in the Jivi indigenous population, Amazonas, Venezuela. Boletin de Malariologia Salud Ambiental. 2010;**50**(2):197-218. Available from: https://ve.scielo.org/scielo.php?script=sci_asttext&pid=S1690-46482010000200004&Ing=es

[10] Memorandum on malaria diagnosis from a WHO meeting. Bulletin of the World Health Organization. 1988;**66**(5):575-594

[11] World Health Organization. Malaria microscopy quality assurance manual, version 2. Geneva: World Health Organization; [Online]. 2016. Available from: https://www.paho.org [Accessed: 07 July 2023]

[12] Kawamoto F. Rapid diagnosis of malaria by fluorescence microscopy whit light microscope and interference filter. Lancet. 1991;**337**(8735):200-202. DOI: 10.1016/0140-6736(91)92159-y

[13] Jelinek T, Grobusch MP, Nothdurft HD. Use of dipstick test for the rapid diagnosis of malaria in nonimmune travelers. Journal of Travel Medicine. 2000;**7**(4):175-179. DOI: 10.2310/7060.2000.00055

[14] Wilson ML. Rapid diagnostic test for malaria. Clinical Infectious Diseases. 2012;**54**(11):1637-1641. DOI: 10.1093/cid/cis228

[15] Abba K, Deeks JJ, Olliaro P, Naing CM, Jackson SM, Takwoingi Y, et al. Rapid diagnostic test for diagnosing uncomplicated P falciparum malaria in endemic countries. Cochrane Database of Systematic Reviews. 2011;**2011**(7):CD008122. DOI: 10.1002/14651858.CD008122.pub2

[16] World Health Organization. Roll Back Malaria & United States. Agency for International Development (2000). New Perspectives; Malaria Diagnosis: Report of a Joint WHO/USAID Informal Consultation, 25-27 October 1999. World Health Organization. Available from: https://apps.who.int/iris/handle/10665/66321 [Accessed: 30 June 2023]

[17] World Health Organization. Regional Office for the Western Pacific. Malaria Rapid diagnosis, making it work, informal consultation on field trials and quality assurance on malaria rapid diagnostic tests. 20-23 January, 2003: Report of the WHO Regional Office for the Western Pacific. 2023. Available from: https://apps.who.int/iris/handle/10665/208030 [Accessed: 30 June 2023]

[18] World Health Organization. Regional Office for the Western Pacific. The use of malaria rapid diagnostic tests. WHO Regional Office for the Western Pacific. 2004. Available from: https://apps.who.int/iris/handle/10665/207715 [Accessed: 25 June 2023]

[19] World Health Organization-Western Pacific Regional Office (WHO-WPRO), USAID/DELIVER PROJECT, Foundation for Innovative New Diagnostics (FIND), Roll Back Malaria Partnership, President's Malaria Initiative (PMI) and UNICEF. Transport, storage and handling of malaria rapid diagnostic tests in central and peripheral storage facilities. Arlington, VA.: USAID/DELIVER PROJECT, Task Order 3; and Manila: WHO-WPRO. July 2009

[20] World Health Organization. Performance of malaria rapid diagnostic tests: Results of WHO product testing of malaria RDTs: Round 8. World Health Organization. License: CC BY-NC-SA 3.0 IGO. 2018. Available from: https://apps.who.int/iris/handle/10665/276190 [Accessed: 23 May 2023]

[21] Beadle C, Long GW, Weiss WR, McElroy PD, Maret SM, Oloo AJ, et al. Diagnosis of malaria by detection of plasmodium falciparum HRP-2 antigen with a rapid dipstick antigen-capture assay. Lancet. 1994;**343**(8897):564-568. DOI: 10.1016/s0140-6736(94)91520-2

[22] De Monbrison F, Gérome P, Chaulet JF, Wallon M, Picot S, Peyron F. Comparative diagnostic performance of two commercial test for malaria in non-endemic area. European Journal of Clinical Microbiology & Infectious Diseases. 2004;**23**(10):784-786. DOI: 10.1007/s10096-004-1202-9

[23] Grobusch MP, Hanscheid T, Zoller T, Jelinet T, Buchard GD. Rapid immunochromatographic malarial antigen detection unreliable for detecting *Plasmodium malariae* and *Plasmodium ovale*. European Journal of Clinical Microbiology & Infectious Diseases. 2002;**21**:818-820. DOI: 10.1007/s10096-002-0831-0

[24] World Health Organization 2017. False-negative RDT results and implications of the new report of histidine-rich protein 2/3 deletions of *P. falciparum*. World Health Organization. 2017. Available from: https://apps.who.

int/iris/handle/10665/ [Accessed: 28 May 2023]

[25] Voller A. The immunodiagnosis of malaria. In: Wernsdorfer WH, Mc Gregor I, editors. Malaria. Principles and Practice of Malariology. Edinburgh: Churchill Livingstone; 1988. pp. 815-827

[26] Farcas GA, Zhong KJ, Lovegrove FE, Graham CM, Kain KC. Evaluation of the Binax NOW ICT test versus polymerase reaction and microscopy for the detection of malaria in returned travelers. American Journal of Tropical Hygiene. 2003;**69**(6):589-592. DOI: 10.4269/ajtmh.2003.69.6.0690589

[27] WHO. WHO Evidence review group on malaria diagnosis in low transmission settings. Meeting report. Geneva: World Health Organization; 2012. Available from: https://www.cdn.who.int/media [Accessed: 29 May 2023]

[28] WHO. Malaria surveillance, monitoring and evaluation: a reference manual. Geneva: World Health Organization. Licence: CC BY-NC-SA 3.0 IGO. 2018. Available from: http://apps.who.int/iris [Accessed: 21 September 2023]

[29] Tarning J, Zongo I, Somé FA, Rouamba N, Parikh S, Rosenthal PJ, et al. Population pharmacokinetics and pharmacodynamics of piperaquine in children with uncomplicated falciparum malaria. Clinical Pharmacological Therapy. 2012;**91**(3):497-505. DOI: 10.1038/clpt.2011.254

[30] Global Antimalarial Resistance Network, (WWARN) DP Study Group. The effect of dosing regimens on the antimalarial efficacy of dihydroartemisinin-piperaquine: A pooled analysis of individual patient data. PLoS Medicine. 2013;**10**(12):e1001564. DOI: 10.1371/annotation/3db421e4-3e27-4442-8092-2ad1b778f371

[31] Cubillos AL, Porras A, Rico A. Efficacy of tafenoquine in the prophylaxis and treatment of Plasmodium vivax malaria, systematic review and meta-analysis. Biomedica;**42**(2):364-377. DOI: 10.7705/biomedica.5988

[32] Padilla JC, Montoya R. Clinical care guidelines for malaria. Infection. 2011;**15**(4):302-323. DOI: 10.1016/s0123-9392(11)70745-7

[33] Cuenca Abruch D, Gómez Johnson VH, Romo López A, Valente-Acosta B. Severe Plasmodium falciparum malaria. AnMed (Mex). 2018;**63**(2):134-137. Available from: www.medigraphic.com/analesmedicos [Accessed: 09 June 2023]

[34] MPPS. PAHO. Treatment guidelines in cases of Malaria. [Internet]. 1st edition. National Malaria Elimination Program. Caracas: Ministerio del Poder Popular para la Salud. 2017:1-118. Available from: https://iris.paho.org/bitstream/handle/10665.2/34490/9789806678057_spa.pdf?sequence=1&is Allowed=y [Accessed: 29 May 2023]

[35] Albrecht-Schgoer K, Lackner P, Schmutzhard E, Baier G. Cerebral malaria: Current clinical and immunological aspects. Frontiers in Immunology. 2022;**13**:863568. DOI: 10.3389/fimmu.2022.863568

[36] World Health Organization. Guidelines for the Treatment of Malaria. 3rd ed. Geneva, Switzerland: World Health Organization, Library Cataloguing-in-Publication Data; 2015. Available from: https://apps.who.int/iris/handle/10665/162441 [Accessed: 26 May 2023]

[37] Esu E, Ea EE, Opie ON, Uwaoma A, Meremikwu MM. Artemether for severe malaria. Cochrane Database of Systematic Reviews. 2014;**2014**(9). CD010678. DOI: 10.1002/14651858. CD010678.pub2 [Accessed: 29 May 2023]

[38] WHO. Guidelines for the Treatment of Malaria. 2nd edition. Geneva: WHO Library Cataloguing-in-Publication Data; 2010. 1-542 pp. Available from: https://www.paho.org/en/node/50095 [Accessed: 30 May 2022]

[39] PAHO. Practical Manual for the Treatment of Severe Malaria. 3rd edition. World Health Organization. Geneva; 2012. 83 p. Available from: https://apps.who.int/iris/bitstream/handle/10665/101443/9789243548524_spa.pdf;jsessionid=E48119EF1D80FF4BC779A23B60DFE046?sequence=1 [Accessed: 07 July 2023]

[40] WHO. Management of severe malaria. Practical manual. 2012. Available from: http://www.mosquito.who.int /docs/hbsm_toc.htlm [Accessed: 05 June 2023]

[41] WHO. Clinical practice guideline. Diagnosis and treatment of malaria. Guideline. 2020;**2020**:40-51. Available from: https://www.who.int/malaria/publications/atoz/9789241549127/en/ [Accessed: 02 June 2023]

[42] Poespoprodjo JR, Burdam FH, Candrawati F, Ley B, Meagher N, Kenangalem E, et al. Supervised versus unsupervised primaquine radical cure for the treatment of falciparum and vivax malaria in Papua, Indonesia: A cluster-randomised, controlled, open-label superiority trial. Lancet Infectious Disease 2022;**22**(3):367-376. DOI: 10.1016/S1473-3099(21)00358-3 [Accessed: 08 June 2023]

[43] Chamma-Siqueira NN, Negreiros SC, Ballard SB, Farias S, Silva SP, Chenet SM, et al. Higher-dose Primaquine to prevent relapse of *Plasmodium vivax* malaria. New England Journal of Medicine 2022;**386**(13):1244-1253. DOI: 10.1056/NEJMoa2104226 [Accessed: 05 July 2023]

Chapter 2

Malaria: Transmission, Diagnosis, Treatment and Prevention in Indonesia

Fitriani Kahar, Yuwono Setiadi, S.Y. Didik Widiyanto, Depri Ardiyansyah and Nurul Qomariyah

Abstract

Malaria is a disease caused by Plasmodium and is characterized by recurrent fever, anemia, and hepatosplenomegaly. There are five species of Plasmodium that can infect humans. *P. falciparum* causes the most deaths, as do *P. vivax*, *P. ovale*, and *P. malariae* which usually cause mild malaria. The aim of this research is to determine the meaning, classification, epidemiology, symptoms, pathogenesis, diagnosis, mode of transmission, prevention, and treatment of malaria. Research method: This research is a descriptive observational study with a literature review design using databases from Google Scholar, accredited national journal Sinta, and reputable international journals such as Scopus, PubMed, Web of Science, and others. The research results show that malaria cases are still high in Indonesia every year. There are several risk factors for malaria such as attitude, behavior, environment, and physical environmental factors where you live, such as (temperature, humidity, livestock pens, houses without screen ventilation, stagnant water, or breeding places). Malaria treatment depends on several factors, including the type of Plasmodium that causes infection, the severity of the disease, and the disease the individual is suffering from. Prevention efforts need to be made by addressing various risk factors for malaria.

Keywords: malaria, transmission, diagnosis, prevention, Indonesia

1. Introduction

The disease caused by Plasmodium is malaria, which is characterized by recurrent fever, anemia, and hepatosplenomegaly. This disease varies from acute to chronic. During the acute phase, attacks of fever sometimes occur. During subsequent chronic stages, there are latent phases separated at relapse in recent times [1]. Malaria is also a health problem that causes death, especially in high-risk groups such as infants, pregnant women, children under five. Malaria also causes anemia and reduces work [2]. Malaria is an endemic disease in Indonesia and affects all components of the blood. The most common complications are anemia and thrombocytopenia. This is a concern of the scientific literature because it is associated with mortality [3]. Indonesia is a tropical country so that malaria is an infectious disease, especially in some areas which are said to be endemic, especially outside Java, such as Jayapura and others [4].

The type of Plasmodium that causes the infection determines the intensity of the symptoms of malaria. Four species of Plasmodium are known: *Plasmodium vivax*, is one of the most common infections causing vuvax or tertian malaria or vivax; *Plasmodium falciparum*, which causes tropical malaria or falciparum malaria, and causes malaria quartana or malriae, nephrotic syndrome and plasmodium ovale which are found in the West Pacific and Africa, resulting in milder outbreaks and frequent outbreaks [5]. There are other species that also cause malaria, that is *Plasmodium knowlesi* [6]. In severe cases will occur malaria cerebral which also has a fatal impact. Nationally, cases have decreased but are still frequently found throughout Indonesia. This disease requires expertise from an appropriate clinical perspective in determining the diagnosis and therapy in patients. Currently, the management of cerebral malaria in Indonesia is guided by the 2017 Malaria Case Management Book [5].

In many countries around the world, malaria is still a public health problem. Even though the Malaria Implementation and Eradication Program has been started since 1959, the mortality and morbidity rates are still high in this country of Indonesia. Every year, 300 million people are attacked and 2–4 million die. Therefore, the Ministry of Health assesses malaria as a very important problem [1].

In 2010 in Indonesia there were 65% of endemic districts where only about 45% of the population in these districts was at risk of contracting malaria. Based on the results of a community survey during 2007–2010, the prevalence of malaria in Indonesia decreased from 1.39% (Riskesdas 2007) to 0.6% (Riskesdas 2010). Meanwhile, based on reports received during 2000–2009, the malaria morbidity rate tended to decrease, namely 3.62 per 1000 population in 2000 to 1.85 per 1000 population in 2009 and 1.96 in 2010. Meanwhile, the death rate due to malaria reached 1.3% [2, 7].

The national prevalence of malaria based on the 2010 Riskesdas results was 0.6% where provinces with API above the national average were West Nusa Tenggara, Maluku, North Maluku, Central Kalimantan, Bangka Belitung, Riau Islands, Bengkulu, Jambi, Central Sulawesi, Gorontalo and Aceh. The highest prevalence rates were found in eastern Indonesia, namely in West Papua (10.6%), Papua (10.1%) and East Nusa Tenggara (4.4%) [2].

Symptoms that patients show upon their arrival at Manado Central Hospital (now known as Bethesda Omolon Hospital and Prof.dr. R.D.Kandou Hospital. In 1993, malaria cases at Bethesda Tomohon Hospital showed objective symptoms of icterus 3.0%, hepatomegaly 43%, splenomegaly 40.7%, and pallor 6.6%.Other common symptoms are vomiting 31–37%, dizziness 75–82%, nausea 74–76%, chills 64–82%, and fever 92–96% [1].

In North Sulawesi, Indonesia, especially in North Sulawesi Hospitals and Health Centers, malaria itself is a disease that is often found. Malaria infection accounts for 9% of hospitalizations, there are 400 cases of mild malaria and 30–40 cases of severe malaria each year, and 6–7 of them die every year. There is a mortality rate from malaria reaching 15.7% in the most common problems that arise are jaundice and kidney failure in Manado City [1].

In South Jayapura District, Indonesia, it is an endemic area with the third highest malaria rate of the 5 districts in Jayapura city. Malaria cases in Jayapura City in 2019 were 28,648 cases with an API of 92.55/1000 population, in 2020 there were 28,075 cases with an API of 89.35/1000 population, while in 2021 there were 30,235 cases with an API of 99.49/1000 population [8].

However, equipment and human resources still greatly influence how quickly and precisely treatment is provided in city and district hospitals. As of December 2009, only a few hospitals, mainly in Manado and Minahasa, had data on malaria patients [1].

1. Problem Formulation

    a. What is the meaning or definition of malaria?

    b. What is the epidemiology of malaria?

    c. How is malaria classified?

    d. What is the scope of malaria?

    e. What are the symptoms of malaria?

    f. What are the risk factors for malaria

    g. What is the pathogenesis of malaria?

    h. What is the immune response to malaria?

    i. What are the diagnoses for malaria?

    j. What are the modes of transmission of malaria?

    k. What are the ways to prevent malaria?

    l. What are the ways to treat malaria?

2. Objective

    a. To understand the meaning of malaria

    b. To understand the epidemiology of malaria

    c. To understand the classification of malaria

    d. To understand the scope of malaria

    e. To understand the symptoms of malaria

    f. To understand the risk factors for malaria

    g. To understand the pathogenesis of malaria

    h. To understand the immune response to malaria

    i. To understand the diagnosis of malaria

j. To understand how malaria is transmitted

k. To understand how to prevent malaria

l. To understand how to treat malaria

3. Benefit

It is hoped that writing this paper will be useful for readers, especially for people in endemic areas to prevent malaria from occurring. Become a source of scientific literature related to malaria.

2. Methodology

Research method: This research is a descriptive observational study with a literature review design with databases from Google Scholar, Sinta accredited national journals, and reputable international journals such as Scopus, Pubmed, Web of Science and others.

3. Result and discussion

3.1 Definition of malaria

Malaria is an infectious disease caused by the bite of the Anopheles mosquito and Plasmodium parasites. Headache, vomiting, chills, fever, and pain in joints and muscles are symptoms of malaria. If treated properly, certain drugs can cure malaria [9]. Malaria is a disease that attacks humans, birds, monkeys and other primates, reptiles and rodents caused by infection with protozoa of the genus Plasmodium. The incidence or transmission of infectious diseases is determined by risk factors/determinants called host, agent and environment [10].

The main cause of this disease is the female Anopheles mosquito which spreads the infection by biting. Anopheles mosquito bites contain parasites in their saliva which enter the blood of the humans they bite. Parasites migrate to the liver, where they mature and reproduce. There are five species of Plasmodium that infect and can infect humans. *P. falciparum* causes the most deaths, as do *P. vivax*, *P. ovale* and *P. malaria* usually cause milder forms of malaria. *P. knowlesi* rarely causes disease in humans. A rapid antigen-based test or a microscopic blood test of a blood sample is usually used to diagnose malaria. Due to cost and complexity, methods for detecting parasite DNA using polymerase chain reactions have not been widely used in areas where malaria is common [9].

3.2 Epidemiology of malaria

Even though there has been a reduction in Annual Parasite Incidence (API) nationally, in areas with high malaria cases the API rate is still very high compared to the national rate, whereas in areas with low malaria cases extraordinary events (KLB) often occur as a result of imported cases. In 2011 the number of reported malaria deaths was 388 case [2].

Information from the World Health Organization (World Health Organization) in 2013 reported that there were 197 million cases of malaria with 548,000 deaths, and 78% of these cases included child deaths under the age of 5 [11]. Furthermore, according to WHO, there were 198 million cases of malaria worldwide in 2014, namely 584. Malaria is widespread in many places around the world, especially in tropical and subtropical regions such as Indonesia. In Indonesia, about 35 percent of the population lives in malaria-prone areas. 584,000 deaths from severe malaria each year. Malaria epidemics occur almost every year in several endemic areas in Indonesia [4]. Areas such as East Nusa Tenggara, West Nusa Tenggara, Maluku, North Maluku, Central Kalimantan, Bangka-Belitung, Riau Islands and Bengkulu are included in the malaria red zone. Next are Jambi, Central Sulawesi, West Sulawesi, Gorontalo and Aceh [4].

Research results related to the prevalence of malaria show that Malaria sufferers were more at the age of 24–35 years, namely as many as 264 sufferers (41.1%), malaria sufferers were more in the female sex as many as 323 people (50.3%), malaria sufferers were more in patients who worked as private employees, namely 410 people (63.9%). More malaria sufferers were found living in urban areas, namely 447 sufferers (69.6%) [12].

Here are some common approaches to treating malaria: Malaria is a disease that is naturally transmitted by pathogens (Plasmodium spp.), definitive hosts (Anopheles spp. and intermediate hosts (humans) [4].

The epidemiological components of malaria consist of: the first pathogen, Plasmodium spp. parasites. Parasites that live in the human body reproduce by consuming red blood cells (RBC), causing anemia in the infected or the host. Second, there are two types of hosts: Humans as intermediate hosts (temporary, because sexual reproduction does not occur) and mosquitoes as definitive hosts (permanent, because sexual reproduction does not occur). Anopheles spp. is a species of mosquito that transmits malaria. However, not all species causes malaria. Plasmodium is spread by malaria, which is bitten by a mosquito (carrier) and then enters the carrier's body via blood cells in various asexual stages. Endemic malaria [4].

3.3 Classification of malaria

Malaria is an infectious disease caused by Plasmodium parasites which can be characterized by fever, hepatosplenomegaly, and anemia. Plasmodium lives and reproduces in human red blood cells. This disease is naturally transmitted through the bite of a female Anopheles mosquito.

Plasmodium species in humans are:

a. *Plasmodium falciparum* (*P. falciparum*).

b. *Plasmodium vivax* (*P. vivax*)

c. *Plasmodium ovale* (*P. ovale*)

d. *Plasmodium malariae* (*P. malariae*)

e. *Plasmodium knowlesi* (*P. knowlesi*)

The most common types of Plasmodium found in Indonesia are *P. falciparum* and *P. vivax*, while *P. malariae* can be found in several provinces, including Lampung, East

Nusa Tenggara, and Papua. P ovale has been found in East Nusa Tenggara and Papua. In 2010 on the island of Borneo it was reported that *P. knowlesi* could infect humans where previously it only infected primates/monkeys and until now [2].

According to Harijanto [13], Malaria is further divided according to its Plasmodium type, including:

3.3.1 Plasmodium falciparum (tropical malaria)

Tropical malaria, also known as tropical falciparum malaria, is the most severe form of malaria. This disease is characterized by anemia, fever, blood parasites, and splenomegaly, often causing complications. The disease lasts 9–14 days. Tropical malaria affects all types of red blood cells caused by *Plasmodium falciparum*. The only Plasmodium species with duplicated nuclear chromatin in the form of a ring or small rings one-third the diameter of a normal red cell. Spread of tropical malaria is classified when *Plasmodium falciparum* infects red cells for life, often resulting in the formation of blood cell parasites that produce multiple protrusions that can adhere to the endothelial lining of capillary walls due to thrombotic occlusion and local ischemia. This infection is more serious than other infections and causes many complications such as cerebral malaria, gastrointestinal disorders and black hemorrhagic fever.

3.3.2 Plasmodium malariae (Kwartama malaria)

Tropozoites of *Plasmodium malariae* which are smaller than *Plasmodium vivax* have more compact or bluer cytoplasm. Mature trophozoites have dark brown to black grains and are often grouped in groups.

3.3.3 Plasmodium ovale (malaria ovale)

Malaria ovale, known as *Plasmodium ovale*, is similar in shape to *Plasmodium malariae*, but the schizont consists of only eight merozoites and has a black mass in the center. Red blood cells infected with *Plasmodium ovale* are usually oval or irregular in shape with a visible ciliated pattern. Of all the types of malaria caused by *Plasmodium ovale*, malaria ovale is the mildest. The incubation period varies from 11 to 16 days, but the latent period can be up to 4 years. Attacks last 3 to 4 days without treatment, rarely more than 10 days, and occur at night.

3.3.4 Plasmodium vivax (tertian malaria)

Plasmodium vivax infection, or tertian malaria, can sometimes affect the young red blood cells, which are larger than normal red blood cells. It resembles *Plasmodium falciparum* in appearance, but vivax trophozoites become amoebae with age. Consists of 12–24 oval merozoites with yellow pigment at the poles. Oval gametocytes occupy almost all of the red blood cells, eccentric chromatin and yellow pigment. Symptoms of this type of malaria last 48 hours as shown in the malaria triad, causing intermittent fever every 4 days, with a peak of fever occurring every 72 hours. Of all the Plasmodium and malaria species that invade the body, tropical malaria is the most important. It is manifested by unstable fever, anemia, splenomegaly, multiple parasites and frequent complications [13].

3.4 Scope malaria

Malaria is a disease in the world, especially in tropical and subtropical regions, the cause of which is the Plasmodium parasite, which is transmitted through the bite of the Anopheles mosquito [14].

The scope of malaria covers several important aspects, including:

1. Geographical breakdown: of 100 countries worldwide, mainly in sub-Saharan Africa, Latin America and parts of Asia. The region where malaria is most common is Africa where malaria is endemic.

2. The Anopheles mosquito is the main cause of malaria. They bite an infected person and then transmit the Plasmodium parasite to other people when they bite.

3. Causes and Types of Parasites: Five different types of Plasmodium cause malaria: *Plasmodium malariae*, *Plasmodium vivax*, *Plasmodium ovale*, *Plasmodium falciparum*, *Plasmodium knowlesi* is the main cause of malaria, the most dangerous of all.

4. Clinical Symptoms: Symptoms of malaria include fever, chills, severe headache, nausea, vomiting and fatigue. If left untreated, malaria can become a life-threatening disease. Prevention: Prevention of malaria involves controlling mosquito vectors through use of insecticide-treated nets, use of antimalarial drugs for prophylaxis, administration of vaccines (such as RTS, S vaccine), and use of mosquito bite prevention measures such as anti-mosquito lotions and repellents

5. Diagnostics and treatment: Diagnosis of malaria involves microscopic examination of blood for the detection of Plasmodium parasites or use of an antigen-based rapid malaria test. Treatment depends on the type of Plasmodium causing the infection and the severity of the disease. Effective antimalarial drugs such as artemisinin-based combination therapy (ACT) are used to treat malaria infection.

6. Social and economic impacts: Malaria has significant social and economic impacts, especially in areas with a high prevalence. Malaria can cause school and work absences, reduced productivity, and a large economic burden on individuals and communities. Tackling the malaria problem requires a comprehensive approach, including vector prevention, effective treatment, access to diagnosis and treatment, and research for the development of more effective vaccines. Global efforts such as vector control campaigns, distribution of insecticide-treated nets, and vaccination initiatives have helped reduce the global burden of malaria. Significant.

7. Genetic Aspects of Malaria: Several genetic factors are the main determinants for child survival in malaria endemic countries. Identification of the genes involved and how they affect the risk of malaria can provide a mechanism for studying the host-parasite relationship. Several gene polymorphisms associated with malaria are Human Red Blood Cell Polymorphisms [15].

3.5 Symptoms of malaria

Manifestations of malaria are fever, anemia and enlargement of the spleen [16].

In people who have been taking antimalarial drugs for prevention, symptoms of malaria may appear later, usually 8 to 25 days after infection. In all types of malaria, the illness is generally flu-like and can mimic sepsis, gastroenteritis, and viruses. Symptoms include: Headache, fever and chills, arthralgia, vomiting, hemolytic anemia, jaundice, urinary hemoglobin, retinal damage and seizures. The main symptoms of malaria are paroxysmal symptoms, including cyclic fever and persistent chills. Then infection with *P. vivax* and *P. ovale* on the second day, called tertiary fever, and every third day, called quarantine fever, with *P. falciparum* can cause recurring fever every 36 to 48 hours or less. One, almost constant fever. *Plasmodium falciparum*, commonly called falciparum malaria, is the main cause of severe malaria. Symptoms of falciparum malaria appear 9 to 30 days after infection. Neurologic symptoms such as nystagmus, postural disturbances, opisthotonos, seizures or coma are common in individuals with cerebral malaria [17].

3.6 Risk factors of malaria

3.6.1 Characteristics of the physical environment

Based on the results of the research that has been carried out, factors that can occur are caused by the roof/wall of the house that is not tightly closed due to the type of wall made of boards or plywood, there is no ceiling, the ventilation of the house does not use gauze, there is a pool of water or *breeding place* such as (gutters, ponds and swamps) as well as houses close to *resting place* or bushes. The factors that have been described will result in the presence of Anopheles sp. mosquitoes if not immediately addressed and corrected.

3.6.2 Behavioral characteristics

Lack of public knowledge about the importance of preventing malaria in their environment and lack of support for malaria cases. It can be concluded that the factors that cause malaria are related to the individual's lack of concern for the environment around his home. Physical environment variables such as the density of the walls of the house, the screens on the ventilation, and the ceilings of the house have relationship with malaria incidence. In addition, behavioral variables such as actions also play a role in the spread of the disease.

To reduce the risk of malaria, people are expected to keep their homes free of mosquitoes by installing tight walls, ceilings and screens for ventilation. In addition, they expect more attention to the environment around the house by adopting environmental management practices, that is, H. save, empty, clean and empty clogged drains and trim bushes.

Malaria control efforts involve environmental management, prevention of mosquito bites, treatment of infected cases, as well as education and community participation. This aims to reduce the presence of mosquito vectors and stop the Plasmodium transmission cycle in the human population [8].

3.7 Pathogenesis of malaria

The rupture of the blood schizont is caused by the release of several antigens and can cause fever in the body. Macrophage cells, monocytes and lymphocytes can be

DOI: http://dx.doi.org/10.5772/intechopen.112982

stimulated by antigens to release cytokine types including Tumor Necrosis Factor. And IL-6 V then enters the hypothalamus, the body's temperature control center. In the four plasmodia it takes a different time for sizogony [2, 18].

Excessive destruction of red blood cells in the malaria parasite is the cause of decreased hemoglobin values, and anemia also occurs due to disturbances in the spinal cord in forming red blood cell [19]. As a result of hemolysis, there is sequestration of erythrocytes in the spleen and other organs, and depression in the bone marrow [16]. In severe cases, cerebral malaria will occur in a febrile patient with decreased consciousness [5]. Cerebral malaria is an acute encephalopathy that meets three criteria, namely coma that cannot be awakened, or coma that persists for >30 minutes after the seizure and is accompanied by *P. falciparum* indicated by a blood smear [20].

Infected or uninfected red blood cells are damaged, causing anemia. Plasmodium ovale and *Plasmodium vivax* infect immature erythrocytes, making up 2% of total erythrocytes, and *P. malariae* only infects mature erythrocytes, making up 1% of total erythrocytes. All types of red blood cells are infected with *Plasmodium falciparum*, so anemia can occur in both acute and chronic infections. Plasmodium lesions are caused by splenic macrophages and lymphocytes, which are reticular endothelial cells. These inflammatory cells enlarge the spleen. Malignant malaria caused by *P. falciparum* has a unique pathogenesis. Once infected with *P. falciparum*, the parasite's red blood cells spread through the capillaries of the body's organs. In addition, the bumps that form on the surface of infected red blood cells contain various *P. falciparum* antigens. Cytokines such as TNF and IL-6, produced by macrophages, monocytes and lymphocytes, activate capillary endothelial cell receptor expression. Cell adhesion occurs when nodules attach to endothelial cell receptors in capillaries. This process causes tissue ischemia due to capillary occlusion. The "asterisk" method - clustering - also supports this inhibition (**Figure 1**) [22].

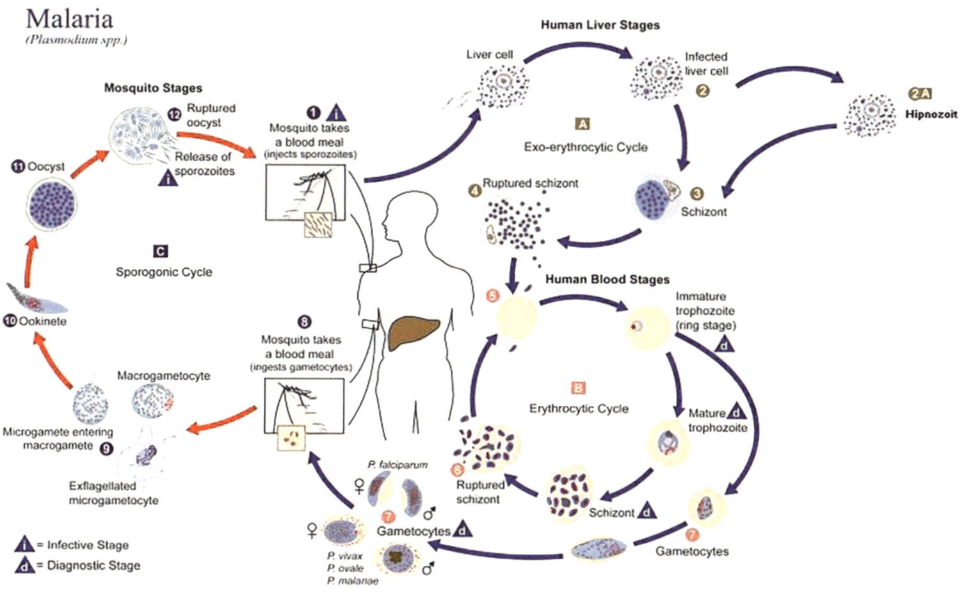

Figure 1.
Plasmodium life cycle in general [21].

3.8 Immune response against malaria

The immune response to malaria infection involves a number of complex mechanisms. When the malaria parasite (Plasmodium) enters the human body through the bite of a vector mosquito, the body's immune system will respond to fight the infection. Following are some of the important stages in the immune response to malaria:

1. Initial stage: After the parasites enter the body, they will enter the liver and reproduce there. During this stage, the initial immune response will involve immune cells such as macrophages and dendritic cells that recognize the parasite and respond by secreting immune-stimulating molecules such as cytokines.

2. Erythrocyte phase: After leaving the liver, the parasite enters red blood cells (erythrocytes) and multiplies there. At this stage, the parasite changes shape and secretes waste products that can trigger an immune response.

3. T cell response: In the fight against malaria infection, T cells, also known as cytotoxic T cells and helper T cells, play an important role. They can recognize parasitic proteins on the surface of infected red blood cells and then act by killing those cells or sending signals to trigger a new immune response.

4. Antibody response: The immune system also produces antibodies to fight parasites. Antibodies are proteins made by plasma cells that can bind to parasites and destroy them, helping to stop them from growing and preventing them from invading more red blood cells.

5. Inflammation: Malaria infection often causes systemic inflammation involving the release of cytokines and other inflammatory molecules. This can cause malaria symptoms such as fever, aches, and malaise.

It is important to note that Plasmodium has the ability to evade or trick the human immune system by changing their protein surface on a regular basis. This allows them to evade detection by the immune system and makes it difficult to develop an effective immune response.

The immune response to malaria can be complex and varies depending on the type of parasite, individual immunity, and other factors. Because of this complexity the development of an effective vaccine for malaria has become a significant challenge in the management of this disease. However, research and efforts are continuing to understand the mechanisms of the immune response and develop effective vaccination strategies [15, 23].

3.9 Diagnosis of malaria

In areas where malaria is rare, the diagnosis of malaria requires a high degree of suspicion, which can be triggered by:

1. Recent travel notes

2. The spleen develops

3. fever

4. Low platelet count

5. Higher than normal blood bilirubin levels in combination with a normal white blood cell count.

Blood smear microscopy or rapid antigen-based test (RDT) is often used to confirm the diagnosis of malaria. In 2010, approximately 165 million meninges were tested for malaria, and microscopy is the most commonly used method of identifying malaria parasites. Despite its widespread use, microscopy has two major drawbacks [2].

In border areas, many testing facilities are not well equipped and the accuracy of results depends on the performance of blood membrane testing kits and the number of parasites in the blood. The sensitivity of blood samples varies between 75 and 90°, up to 50% under optimal conditions. Commercially available RDTs are often more accurate than blood films in predicting the presence of malaria parasites, but their diagnostic sensitivity and specificity vary widely between manufacturers and cannot be determined. Any healthy person who has traveled to a malaria endemic area should be suspected of having malaria and examined where tests are available. In places where laboratory diagnostic tests cannot be performed, the use of pre-existing fever as an indication for treatment of malaria has become widespread. As a result, the popular notion that "fever is synonymous with malaria if proven otherwise" has spread. Malaria over diagnosis and poor non-malarial therapy limit this approach, consume limited resources, reduce trust in the health system and increase drug resistance. Although assays that rely on polymerase chain reaction have been developed, their complexity has prevented their widespread use in areas where malaria is common. Increased resistance to polymerase chains has been developed, but because of its complexity it is not widespread in areas where malaria is common [2].

3.10 Transmission of malaria

The determinants of malaria transmission are divided into two broad categories. First, the factors that have a direct effect, the average mosquito bites humans in a day, the average Plasmodium gametocytes in the population, the length of the sporogonic cycle in the mosquito's body, the average daily survival rate of mosquitoes. Second, indirect factors, including environment and climate, rainfall, drought, management of the artificial environment, changes in vector biting patterns, air temperature, humidity, importation of malaria parasites through population movements and migration of non-immune populations [24].

One of the ways that malaria can be transmitted is by the bite of a vector mosquito infected with Plasmodium. Here are some ways of transmitting malaria:

1. Anopheles mosquito bites: The main cause of malaria is the bite of the Anopheles mosquito. When a mosquito bites a person infected with malaria, Plasmodium in their blood can enter the mosquito's body. When the mosquito bites another person, Plasmodium infects the person bitten and causes a malaria infection.

2. Blood transfusion: In rare cases, malaria can also be transmitted by blood transfusion. When a person with malaria donates blood, Plasmodium in the blood can infect the recipient.

3. The use of syringes that are contaminated with blood containing Plasmodium can also be a source of malaria transmission. This can happen if needles are used simultaneously by people infected with malaria and other people without adequate sterilization procedures.

4. Perinatal Transmission: It is possible for malaria to be transmitted from a pregnant woman who is infected with malaria to her baby during pregnancy or childbirth. This is known as perinatal transmission [4].

3.11 Prevention of malaria

Efforts to eradicate malaria in Indonesia have not achieved optimal results due to several factors such as the prevalence of malaria mosquitoes, the high number of cases, human resources, costs and infrastructure. Therefore, the best course of action is to prevent and stop the spread of the parasite. Many efforts can be made to prevent and eradicate the spread of malaria parasite [25].

Methods for preventing mosquito bites are particularly important in high prevalence areas. It is recommended to wear long sleeves and long pants when going out, especially at night, in rural or suburban areas with lots of rice fields, swamps or fish ponds (ideal breeding grounds for malaria-carrying mosquitoes).

Efforts to reduce morbidity and mortality are carried out through a malaria eradication program whose activities include early diagnosis, prompt and appropriate treatment, and vector surveillance and control in terms of public education and understanding of environmental health, all of which are aimed at breaking the chain of malaria transmission.

Resistance cases of malaria parasites to chloroquine were first discovered in East Kalimantan in 1973 for *P. falciparum*, and in 1991 for *P. vivax* in Nias. Since 1990, cases of resistance have been reported to have spread in all provinces in Indonesia. In addition, there have also been reports of resistance to Sulfadoxine-pyrimethamine (SP) in several places in Indonesia. This situation can increase the morbidity and mortality of malaria. Therefore, to overcome this problem of resistance (multiple drug resistance) and the existence of new anti-malarial drugs that are more patent, the government has recommended drugs of choice to replace chloroquine and SP, namely a combination of artemisinin derivatives with other anti-malarial drugs which are commonly referred to as Artemisinin based [2].

3.12 Treatment of malaria

Treatment of malaria depends on several factors, including the type of Plasmodium causing the infection, the severity of the disease, and the individual's health condition [9].

1. Antimalarial drugs: Antimalarial drug therapy is the main step in the treatment of malaria. Several types of drugs are used including:

- Artemisinin-based combination therapy (ACT) This is the standard treatment for malaria caused by *Plasmodium falciparum*. ACT combines artemisinin compounds with other antimalarial drugs to treat infections.

- Chloroquine: Chloroquine is usually used to treat malaria caused by *Plasmodium malariae*, *Plasmodium vivax* and *Plasmodium ovale*. However, many areas of the world report resistance to chloroquine, limiting its use. Other drugs: There are other antimalarial drugs used in the treatment of malaria, such as mefloquine, doxycycline, atovaquone/proguanil, and kinin. The choice of drug depends on the type of Plasmodium and the level of resistance in the affected area [26].

2. Supportive therapy. In severe cases of malaria, supportive therapy may be required. This involves monitoring and managing symptoms such as high fever, dehydration, electrolyte disturbances, anemia, and organ dysfunction. In some cases, hospitalization may be required for more intensive monitoring and adequate treatment.

3. Prevention of complications: Malaria can cause serious complications, such as severe anemia, respiratory problems, kidney failure and neurological disorders. Prevention and treatment of these complications is also an important part of malaria management.

It is important to note that antimalarial drug resistance is becoming an increasingly serious problem in some areas. Therefore, it is important to follow medication recommendations and consult a doctor who is experienced in treating malaria. In addition to treatment, prevention of malaria is essential, including the use of insecticide-treated nets and the prophylactic use of antimalarial drugs for those living in or traveling to remote areas. Use of mosquito repellents and control of mosquito vectors through eradication programs or the use of chemical insecticides (**Table 1**) [9].

4. Conclusions

Tackling the malaria problem requires a comprehensive approach that includes vector prevention, effective treatment, access to diagnosis and treatment, and research to develop more effective vaccines. Global efforts such as vector control campaigns, distribution of insecticide-treated bed nets and vaccination initiatives have helped reduce the global burden of malaria.

There are several risk factors for the occurrence of malaria such as attitudes, behavior, environment and physical environmental factors of residence such as (temperature, humidity, presence of cattle pens, the house is not ventilated through gauze, there are stagnant water or breeding grounds. Treatment of Malaria Treatment of malaria depends on several factors, including the type of Plasmodium that causes the infection, the severity of the disease and the individual's illness. It is necessary to carry out prevention efforts by addressing various risk factors for malaria to prevent cases of malaria. One way to prevent and overcome malaria is to improve individual and environmental sanitation.

No	Researcher	Research title	Results	Discussion
1	Ragil Setiabudi, [27]	Systematic Review: Risk of Malaria as an Infectious Disease in Indonesia	Based on the similarity of variables between researchers, there are 21 significant risk factors statistically, namely the presence of mosquito breeding places, without screens/barriers on ventilation of the house, not using mosquito coils, presence of bushes, presence of puddles water, presence of paddy fields, presence of ditches/gutches, presence of animal cages, poor housekeeping, house walls not tight, no ceiling, construction of non-permanent house floors, frequent activities outside the home at night, not using mosquito nets when sleeping, hanging clothes in the house, not using pesticides/insecticides, not using mosquito repellant/topical repellant, low education, income below the minimum wage, non-compliance with taking medication, malnutrition status with an average OR = 5.30. Minimum value OR = 0.26 and maximum value OR = 16.92. There are only two protective factors, namely frequent using mosquito nets on the bed (OR = 0.26) and having a ceiling (OR = 0.69).	Risk factors for malaria incidence in Indonesia which means statistically there are 21 namely the presence of mosquito breeding places, without gauze/barrier on ventilation house, do not use mosquito coils, the presence of bushes, the presence of standing water, there are rice fields, there are ditches/ditches, existence of animal cages, cleanliness bad house, the walls of the house are not tight, no ceiling house, construction house floors are not permanent, often outdoor activities at night did not use mosquito nets at the time sleep, hang clothes inside house, do not use pesticides/insecticides, do not use repellant/repellent topical medication mosquitoes, primary education, income in below the minimum wage, non-compliance taking medication, poor nutritional status. The average OR for the incidence of Malaria is 5.30 The protective factor for the occurrence of Malaria is the frequent use of mosquito nets on the bed and the presence of a ceiling

DOI: http://dx.doi.org/10.5772/intechopen.112982

No	Researcher	Research title	Results	Discussion
2	Utami, Tya Palpera Hasyim, Hamzah Kaltsum, Ummi Dwifitri, Uthu Meriwati, Yanti Yuniwarti, Yuniwarti Paridah, Yusro Zulaiha, Zulaiha [28]	Risk Factors Causing Malaria in Indonesia: Literature Review	Malaria is still a disease with high cases in Indonesia for everyone the year. Factors that cause malaria in Indonesia consist of factors people's behavior and attitudes (nighttime activities, use of anti-inflammatory drugs) mosquitoes and use of mosquito nets), environmental factors and the physical environment place of residence (presence of livestock pens, presence of bushes, presence of watery rice fields, temperature, humidity, presence of wires on ventilation, the condition of the ceiling of the residence, and the density of the walls of the house). One of ways to prevent and combat malaria by increasing individual and environmental sanitation.	Community behavior and attitudes Public awareness can be seen from the preventive measures taken such as [1] The habit of staying out late at night, [2] Carrying out environmental health activities, [3] Using mosquito nets. The purpose of using mosquito nets while sleeping is to limit mosquitoes that are infected with bite healthy people and healthy mosquitoes bite sick people, [4] Using household mosquito repellents. Household insecticides are anti-mosquito products that are often used by the community, such as mosquito coils and anti-mosquito sprays [5] Use of mosquito repellents [6]. Use of Body Cover, [7] Installation of Gauze Wire on window doors to prevent mosquitoes from entering the house Environmental factor Physical environmental factors of the house (temperature, humidity, the presence of wires on the ventilation, the existence of the ceiling of the house, and the density of the walls of the house). The spread of malaria depends on the interaction between the carrier agent, the host and the environment. The environment that plays a role in the bionomic development of mosquitoes is the physical environment and the biological environment. The environment has a major influence on the incidence of malaria. The existence of brackish water lakes, stagnant water in forests, rice fields, fish ponds, clearing of forests and mining in an area will increase because these places are places where malaria mosquitoes spread.

No	Researcher	Research title	Results	Discussion
3	Suwito Hadi, Upik Kesumawati Sigit, Singgih H Sukowati, Dan Supratman [29]	Climate Relations, Density Anopheles mosquito and Genesis Malaria disease	*A. sundaicus* mosquito is a type of mosquito that is influential in Rajabasa Subdistrict and Weather Mirror Field have no relationship means the number of Anopheles mosquitoes.	The Rajabasa sub-district found 10 species of Anopheles that came into contact with humans, namely *A. sundaicus*, *A. vagus*, *A. tessellatus*, *A. aconitus*, *A. subpictus*, *A. annularis*, *A. kochi*, *A. minimus*, *A. barbirostris* and *A. maculatus*. The Padangcermin sub-district found eight species of Anopheles that came into contact with humans, namely *A. sundaicus*, *A. subpictus*, *A. barbirostris*, *A. kochi*, *A. aconitus*, *A. tessellatus*, *A. vagus* and *A. hyrcanus* group. The *A. sundaicus* mosquito is the dominant species in Rajabasa and Padang-mirror sub-districts, as shown by the very high number of bites per person per hour (MHD) compared to other species. The increase in air humidity and rainfall is directly proportional to the increase in mosquito density. Rainfall has a significant relationship with mosquito density Anopheles, while the density of Anopheles mosquitoes has a significant relationship with malaria cases 1 month later.

No	Researcher	Research title	Results	Discussion
4	Permadani, Yudea Patungo, Viertianingsih Nompo, R [30]	literature Review: Community Behavior in Malaria Prevention	Research result This literature shows that the level of knowledge, the attitudes and actions of the community in the prevention of malaria are still low so that it affects the low malaria prevention behavior such as the use of mosquito nets in the community and use of mosquito repellents and installation of wire netting on house ventilation. Public awareness in preventing malaria is shown in behavior community through keeping the environment clean, insecticide-treated mosquito nets, wire netting on ventilation houses, counseling health workers and the use of anti-mosquito drugs. This behavior delivers	**Environmental hygiene** The environment is very important in the prevention of malaria. The areas where people live mostly have bushes around the house, some people also live near rivers where there is still a lot of plastic waste scattered which causes mosquitoes to breed. The existence of malaria mosquitoes in an area is very dependent on the environment, where they are often found mosquito breeding around terraced rice fields and irrigation canals. Another effort is to do 3 M (draining, closing and burying) Draining is cleaning a place that is often used as a water reservoir such as a bathtub, water bucket, drinking water reservoir, refrigerator water reservoir and others. **Wire mesh on house ventilation** Installation of wire netting in the ventilation holes of the house is one step to limit the entry of malaria-transmitting mosquitoes into the house. **Mosquito repellent** The most widely used types of mosquito repellents are the types of mosquito coils and anti-mosquito lotions. People who are used to using mosquito repellents while sleeping or outside the home are aware of the dangers of malaria **Health worker education** Apart from installing ventilation screens at home, health workers very rarely conduct counseling so that not much information is obtained by the community about the incidence of malaria

No	Researcher	Research title	Results	Discussion
5.	Fitriani Kahar, Djoko Priyatno, Beatrix Marta Meo [31]	Study Of Erythrocyte Index In Malaria Positive Diagnosis Patients	Research on examining the value of the erythrocyte index in patients with a positive diagnosis of malaria using the manual method can be concluded that there is an MCV that is less than normal is 50%, normal is 50% and which is more than normal is 0%. MCH less than is 35%, normal 65%, and more than normal 0%. MCHC that is less than normal and more than normal is 0% while the normal is 100%.	In addition, a definite diagnosis of malaria is by microscopic examination and finding malaria parasites in the blood and supported by clinical symptoms in patients. On positive patient blood smears malaria, visible differences in blood cells red and forms of the malaria parasite. Next, check the quantity erythrocyte and hematocrit values. Malaria infection is one of the main infectious diseases that occur in the world that causes infection in humans humans with fever periodic occurrence of fever due to infection from malaria parasites (including protozoa) transmitted by Anopheles mosquitoes. Manifestations of malaria are fever, anemia and spleen enlargement. The life cycle of the parasite takes place in humans and in mosquitoes.

Table 1.
Table of literature research results.

DOI: http://dx.doi.org/10.5772/intechopen.112982

Acknowledgements

Thank you to the Poltekkes Kemenkes Semarang who have contributed invaluable in writing this scientific paper, and to the team that has assisted in collecting data in this study.

Funding

Nil.

Conflict of interest

No conflicts of interest are disclosed by the authors.

Notes/thanks/other declarations

The concept of this paper was developed by F.K, Y.S, S.Y.D.W, D.A, and NQ, who also wrote the script. The final manuscript submitted has been read and approved by all authors.

Author details

Fitriani Kahar[1*], Yuwono Setiadi[2], S.Y. Didik Widiyanto[1], Depri Ardiyansyah[3] and Nurul Qomariyah[1]

1 Department of Health Analyst, Ministry of Health Polytechnic, Semarang, Indonesia

2 Department of Nutrition, Ministry of Health Polytechnic Semarang, Indonesia

3 Department of Environmental Health, Health Polytechnic Ministry of Health, Semarang, Indonesia

*Address all correspondence to: fitrianikahar555@gmail.com

IntechOpen

© 2023 The Author(s). Licensee IntechOpen. This chapter is distributed under the terms of the Creative Commons Attribution License (http://creativecommons.org/licenses/by/3.0), which permits unrestricted use, distribution, and reproduction in any medium, provided the original work is properly cited.

References

[1] Purwanto DS, Ottay RI. Profile of malaria disease in inpatients at the regional general hospital in Bitung city. Journal of Biomedicine. 2013;**3**(3):172-178. Available from: file:///C:/Users/Amir/Downloads/jm_biomedik,+6.+Nu+Profil+penyakit+malaria+(7hal).pdf

[2] Republic of Indonesia Ministry of Health. Regulation of the minister of health of the Republic of Indonesia No. 5 of 2013 concerning guidelines for malaria management. In: Regulation of the Minister of Health of the Republic of Indonesia. Jakarta: RI Ministry of Health; 2013. pp. 5-62. Available from: www.djpp.depkumham.go.id

[3] Natalia D. The role of platelets in the pathogenesis of malaria. Majalah Kedokteran Andalas. 2015;**37**(3):219

[4] Hakim L. Malaria: Epidemiology and diagnosis. Aspirator. 2011;**3**(2):107-116. Available from: https://media.neliti.com/media/publications-test/53932-malaria-epidemiologi-dan-diagnosis-cad38e4c.pdf

[5] Mawuntu AHP. Cerebral malaria. Journal of Synapse. 2018;**1**(3):1-21

[6] Singh B, Daneshvar C. Human infection and detection of plasmodium knowlesi. Clinical Microbiology Reviews. 2013;**26**:165-184

[7] WHO. World Malaria Report 2005 [Internet]. WHO. 1AD. Available from: https://www.malariaconsortium.org/userfiles/file/Malariaresources/WMReport_lr.pdf

[8] Madayanti S, Raharjo M, Purwanto H. Risk factors affecting malaria incidents in the South Jayapura district, Jayapura city. Journal of Indonesian Environmental Health. 2022;**21**(3):358-365

[9] Supranelfy Y, Oktarina R. Description of malaria disease prevention behavior in South Sumatra (advanced analysis of Riskesdas 2018). Balaba J R & D for Control of Animal-Based Diseases of Banjarnegara. 2021;**17**(1):19-28. Available from: http://ejournal2.bkpk.kemkes.go.id/index.php/blb/article/view/3556

[10] Sitepu R, Lukito A, Tarigan E. Determinant analysis of malaria disease in Kutambaru District in 2017. Journal of Medicine and Health Sciences. 2018;**5**(3):165-173. Available from: https://ejurnalmalahayati.ac.id/index.php/kesehatan/article/view/165-173/pdf

[11] World Health Organization. World Malaria Report. WHO Global Malaria Programme; 2012. p. 195. [Internet]. ISBN: 9789241564533. Available from: http://www.who.int/malaria/world_malaria_report_2012/en/, https://www.who.int/publications/i/item/9789241564533

[12] Alim A, Adam A, Dimi B. Prevalence of malaria based on socio demographic characteristics. Journal of Health Sciences. 2020;**19**(1):4-9

[13] Harijanto P. Malaria, Epidemiology, Pathogenesis, Clinical Manifestations and Treatment. Jakarta: EGC; 2000. Available from: http://elib.unisa-bandung.ac.id/index.php?p=show_detail&id=4309

[14] Ngambut K, Sila O. Environmental factors and community behavior about malaria in East Kupang District, Kupang regency. National Public Health Journal. 2013;**7**(6):271-278. Available from: https://jurnalkesmas.ui.ac.id/kesmas/article/view/37

[15] Wahyuni S. Gene polymorphism in malaria. Averrous Journal Medical and Health Malikussaleh. 2018;**2**(1):35.

Available from: https://ojs.unimal.ac.id/averrous/article/view/411/335

[16] Fitriany J, Sabiq A. Malaria. Journal of Averrous. 2018;**4**:2

[17] Selvia D. Leaving the house at night and using insecticide nets for malaria in Lempasing village. Journal of Health Sciences. 2019;**1**(2):88-95. Available from: https://salnesia.id/jika/article/view/29

[18] Miller LH, Baruch DI, Marsh K, Doumbo OK. The pathogenic basis of malaria. Pathogesis Basis Malar. 2002;**415**(6872):673-679. Available from:. DOI: 10.1038/415673a

[19] Isnaini H, Kristinawati E, Rohmi A. Hemoglobin levels and platelet counts on malaria positivity at the Meninting and Gunung sari health centers in West Lombok. Jurnal Analis Medika Biosains (JAMBS) [Journal of Medical Analysts Biosciences]. 2018;**5**(2):107-113. Available from: http://jambs.poltekkes-mataram.ac.id/index.php/home/article/view/114

[20] Husna M, Prasetyo BH. Review of biomolecular aspects and updates on cerebral malaria therapy. MNJ. 2016;**2**(2):79-88

[21] CDC. Malaria: Biology. Centers For Disease Control and Prevention (CDC); 2020. p. 1. Available from: https://www.cdc.gov/malaria/about/biology/index.html

[22] Dinata A. Plasmodium and the Life Cycle of the Malaria Parasite (World Malaria Day Records). Indonesia: Publikasi; 2022. p. 1. Available from: https://litbangkespangandaran.litbang.kemkes.go.id/plasmodium-dan-daur-hidup-parasit-malaria-catatan-hari-malaria-sedunia/

[23] Mukh S. The role of immune factors and protein profiles in research and development of irradiated malaria vaccines. Biosaintifika: Journal of Biology & Biology Education. 2014;**6**(1):8-17

[24] Solikhah S. Identification of malaria vectors. Public Health National Public Health Journal. 2013;7(9):402-407

[25] WHO. Future Malaria Treatment. South-East Asia Indonesia: WHO; 2021. Available from: https://www.who.int/indonesia/news/campaign/world-malaria-day-2021/pengobatan-malaria-masa-depan

[26] Guerin PJ, Olliaro P, Nosten F, Druilhe P, Ramanan Laxminarayan Binka F, Kilama WL, et al. Malaria: Current status of control, diagnosis, treatment, and a proposed agenda for research and development. Lancet. 2002;**2**(9):567-573. Available from: https://www.thelancet.com/journals/laninf/article/PIIS1473-3099(02)00372-9/fulltext

[27] Setiabudi R. Risk factors for malaria as an infectious disease. Medicines Journal Ilm Health Sciences. 2016;**14**(1):53-64

[28] Utami TP, Hasyim H, Kaltsum U, Dwifitri U, Meriwati Y, Yuniwarti Y, et al. Risk factors causing malaria in Indonesia: Literature review. Journal of Surya Medicine. 2022;7(2):96-107

[29] Suwito HUK, Sigit SH, Sukowati DS. Relationship of climate, density of anopheles mosquitoes and malaria disease incidence. Journal Entomology Indonesia. 2010;**7**(1):42-53

[30] Permadani Y, Patungo V, Nompo RS. Literature review: Community behavior in preventing malaria. Sentani Nursing Journal. 2022;**5**(2798-5075):21-28. Available from: https://ejournal.stikesjypr.ac.id/index.php/snj

[31] Kahar F, Priyatno D, Meo BM. Study of erythrocyte index in patients with positive diagnosis of malaria. Journal of Sololipu Community Media Akad and Community Community. 2020;**20**(2):175-182

Section 2

Malaria Transmission

Chapter 3

One Health Perspective of Malaria Transmission

Jonas Bedford Danquah and Jennifer Afua Afrifa Yamoah

Abstract

Global efforts towards malaria control and elimination are promising. Despite this, current alterations in transmission continue to modify and frustrate such effort. In 2020 and 2021, malaria transmissions increased significantly. While 2021 showed a decline in malaria deaths by 6000 (1%), the numbers were still 51,000 (9%) higher than malaria deaths in 2019. Two-thirds of the contributing factors were attributed to the COVID-19 pandemic, thus demonstrating the capability of future pandemics and zoonotic diseases to stagger or derail earned achievements towards malaria elimination. Compounded by zoonotic and environmental factors that promote malaria transmission, there will be a need for relevant modelling and an update on current and past disease distribution information and will also be required to shape policy actions and to improve public health decision-making on malaria. These will help strengthen the evidence for the adoption of relevant implementation strategies to aid the 2030 vision of eliminating malaria a reality.

Keywords: zoonotic malaria, environmental transmission, non-human malaria, endemicity, pandemic

1. Introduction

Malaria is an ancient disease of public health concern, which has scourged and threatened humanity for many centuries till today. The nemesis of it was estimated to be over 400 million deaths recorded globally within the 20th century alone [1]. Archaeological artefacts and relics of clay tablets, papyrus, religious and medical texts, parasite DNA detections in mummified remains, modelled ancient seasonal and climatic indicators are chest of trove suggesting that the disease has since been known perhaps during the Palaeolithic and Neolithic era [2–6]. The means of disease transmission remained elusive until the discovery of the malaria parasite by Charles Alphonse Laveran in 1880 and the related transmission vector by Sir Ronald Ross in 1897.

Preceding Laveran and Ross's findings are remarkable leads. These include a 270 BC Chinese canonic account in the "*Huangdi Neijing*" describing periodic fevers associated with enlarged spleen and prescriptions of Qinghaosu (Artemisinin) for treatment [7–10]. The Greeks also linked malaria with swampy and marshy environments [1, 9]. Further observed cases of tertian and quartan fevers reported by Hippocrates (460–370 BC), Celsius and Galen were high during the late summer and autumn seasons and coincided with the appearance of Sirius – the dog star illustrated by Homer in his epic [5, 9, 11, 12]. Gleaning from the Greeks, theories of Miasma emerged, with the Romans also attributing the disease transmission to either drinking marsh water or another positing the cause to be due to inhaled vapours from marshes [1, 9, 13]. During these periods Robert Koch introduced the Koch postulate in the era of the germ theory. This led to a new wave of infectious disease research meant to identify and relate pathogens such as the malaria parasites to the respective diseases.

Leveraging on the advances made in infectious disease research and the observation that there were other low malaria transmission areas with no swamp or marsh, Laveran observed and described the malaria parasite from the blood of malaria patients in Algeria in 1880 [14–16]. His initial finding was first met with scepticism not until 1896 when he further produced inevitable proof, which corrected the erroneous competing ideas of Ettore Marchiafava and Augusto Celli's attribution of the disease to a bacterium they named *Bacillus malaria* [13, 14, 17]. Entry of *Plasmodium* species into humans now became a subject of interest with the initial hypothesis suggesting a possible involvement of Mosquitoes as mooted by Sir Patrick Manson.

Inspired by the work of Laveran and Manson, Ross started his work to prove Manson's hypothesis at Secunderabad in India [18–20]. When confronted with a shortage of experimental samples after his posting to Calcutta, Ross resorted to the use of avian malaria models for his studies and this largely gave clues to his discovery [14, 19, 20]. Ross in 1897 established the involvement of mosquitoes in the transmission cycle and described the sexual developmental stages of *Plasmodium* within the mosquito [18–20]. This disproved the aspect of Manson's hypothesis, which suggested that the parasite-infected via an oral route through drinking water infested with the malaria parasite. It further disproved the postulate that transmission was by inhaling bad air from swamps [14, 19, 20]. Grassi and co-workers in 1898 also established that human malaria is solely transmitted by the female *Anopheles* mosquito [18–20]. Building on Ross' publications the team characterised the mosquito species (*Anopheles claviger*), which was involved in the transfer of the *Plasmodium* parasite and also described the sporogony stage of human *Plasmodium* [18–20].

2. Global malaria trends in pre- and post-COVID era

Past accounts of malaria and its transmissions were dealt with on a local basis and the clarity we have today was a bit blurred in those times. Increased knowledge of malaria and a much-coordinated global effort garnered in the battle against malaria within the early 1900s are yielding fruit today. However, this global effort has been met with various successes and challenges, that have reshaped previous strategies designed to meet milestone targets set from the period of millennium development goals (MDG) through to the current sustainable development goals (SDG). The success of the new wave of revolution against malaria is the disease eliminated in Europe and certain regions of the world as well as a massive decline in deaths due to the disease. In 2021, COVID-19 was estimated to have accounted for two-thirds of the challenges that were raised to have affected targeted milestones for malaria making it important to review the period in question.

Considering the global report on malaria from 2019 to 2022, the burden of malaria is still high showing an increase of 16 million more malaria cases reported in the post-COVID era than in the pre-COVID period (2018) [21]. A global outlook on malaria case fatality rate (CFR) shows a moderately stable CFR of between 0.0% and 0.3% during the pre- and post-COVID period as illustrated in **Figure 1** for all the WHO regions. The trend further reflects a marginal decline in mortality from 625,000 in 2020 to 619,000 in 2021 [21]. Despite the slight decline in deaths for 2022, the numbers were still approximately 9% higher than malaria deaths reported during the pre-COVID period in 2018 (567,000) [21].

Malaria milestone targets set in 2015 are almost midway through the end date [21]. These targets were not entirely met by most of the WHO-endemic regional blocs with the exception of the South East Asia region, which was resilient through the period under purview. The worst-case scenario was observed for the Africa region, which accounted for 94% of the global cases of malaria in 2021 with an average estimated 0.3% case fatality rate (**Figure 1**). Of the mortalities reported in 2021 within the Africa bloc, 80% occurred in children under the age of 5 with Case incidence (cases per 1000 population at risk) and mortality targets being 45 and 75% off track respectively to the baseline target set for the Global technical strategy for malaria (GTS) for 2020 [21]. South East Asia region with most of its cases reported from India (79%) and the Eastern Mediterranean regions accounted for 2.5% each of the global cases of malaria. Western Pacific and American regions also contributed 0.6 and 0.2%, respectively (**Figure 1**) [21].

The recent COVID-19 pandemic in 2019, posited to have a zoonotic origin led to the enforcement of various restrictions. This did not only affect global commerce and international travel activities but also impacted health services and deliveries of which malaria is a part. Amid existing robust strategies in place for the elimination of malaria, COVID-19 has demonstrated the potency of potential future zoonotic pandemics to impinge on healthcare delivery and malaria milestone targets towards 2030. The panacea is to expand the strategic scope to include animal and environmental health mitigation strategies, which will demand open discussions and improve upon resilience in the fight against malaria.

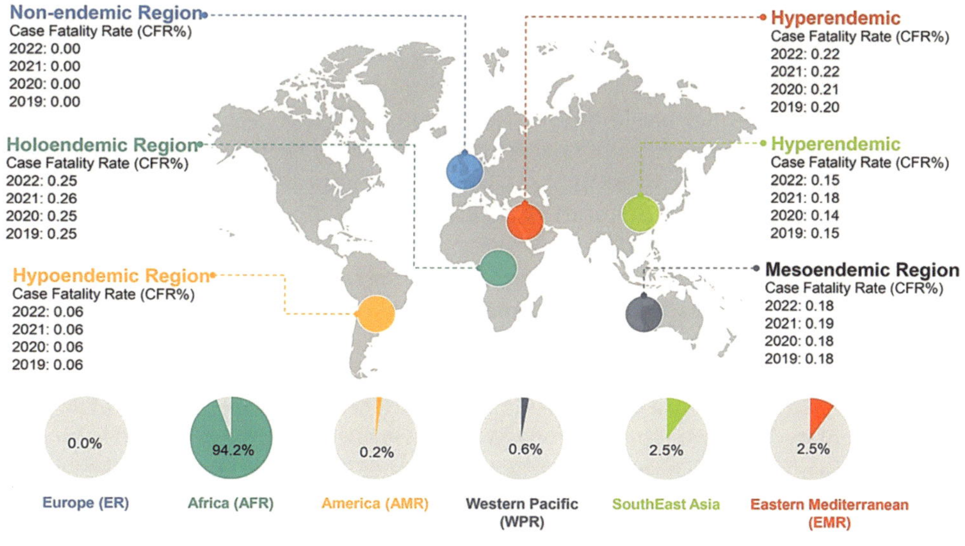

Figure 1.
Malaria burden in pre- and post-COVID period across WHO regions (author construct: 2023).

3. Human malaria transmissions

Early studies on malaria have identified various forms of malaria and possible routes of entry used by the *Plasmodium* parasite to invade the host. This includes asymptomatic forms, congenital and neonatal malaria, cerebral malaria and imported malaria cases. These can be transmitted directly by a female *Anopheles* species or through parenteral transmissions including those acquired through blood transfusion, pricks from sharps and organ transplantation routes. Malaria infections irrespective of the route of entry in humans have been associated with unique cyclical fevers which were known from the past. These fevers could be described as tertian, quartan, and quotidian [5, 22–27].

Each of these fevers, with their severity and other unique clinical presentations, has been well characterized and known today to be associated with specific *Plasmodium* species [5, 23, 27–30]. Four main human *Plasmodium* species and a zoonotic species *Plasmodium knowlesi* are currently known to cause the disease in humans [5, 23, 27–30]. The identification of these *Plasmodium* species and their related fevers was therefore a remarkable breakthrough that has aided our better understanding of human malaria transmission today. While *P. knowlesi*, is currently the only known parasite species associated with quotidian malaria parasite-related fevers [5, 23, 27–30]. Tertian malaria on the other hand, which may exist in benign or malignant forms are known to be the most abundant indicating a high host and vector preference for members (*Plasmodium* species) of the tertian group [5, 23, 27–30].

4. Non-human malaria transmission

Non-human *Plasmodium* infections have played a significant role in unravelling the puzzle of human malaria transmissions. Non-human infections can be transmitted directly through the bite of a vector or congenital means to a non-human susceptible species. Laboratory transmissions to non-human vertebrate models are sustained and made possible parenterally using cell cultures or blood infected with the parasite [26, 31–34]. Moreover, cell-to-cell based transmissions are also made possible in cell cultures with studies investigating parasite development, drug resistance, host response, and parasite-host interactions benefiting immensely from such culture-based and animal-based model transmissions [26, 31–34]. Currently, more than 250 species of *Plasmodium* parasites are known today to infect various vertebrate hosts, including humans, non-human primates (Prosimian, Apes, old and new world monkeys), birds, reptiles, rodents and ungulates among other mammals [31, 35].

The use of transmission models or other vertebrate models, therefore serves as an alternative for complementary studies on confounding factors limiting malaria experimentations in humans [31, 34]. Ross and other independent workers pioneered research on avian malaria in 1897, this led to the discovery of various avian-specific *Plasmodium* species that are useful for laboratory studies [18–20]. This included studies on malaria transmission in different bird species and the identification of avian-specific vectors that are competent in the transfer of different *Plasmodium* species across susceptible bird species [19, 36]. The avian group served as a forerunner host model to unveil the sporogonic developmental stages of human malaria parasites within the mosquito vector.

Rodent malaria parasites, after their discovery in 1940, have also played a significant role in our current knowledge of malaria transmission over time [32, 37, 38]. This spans from basic laboratory research to iterative ones in both immunological and malaria vaccine candidate tests. The rodent *Plasmodium P. berghei ANKA* has been found useful as a model for learning about cerebral malaria. Rodents are smaller in size requiring less housing space with a faster perpetuation time and like their bird counterparts they produce more offspring than most primates. Laboratory adaptable strains of rodent *Plasmodium* transmissions offer a comparative evaluation of malaria within a small controlled environmental condition.

Plasmodium transmission patterns among primates are similar to human malaria infections. Gleaning from the genetic relatedness of humans with great apes and other members of the monkey family, Laveran became the first to observe *Plasmodium pitheci* in the blood of orangutans in 1905. Further works on great apes in Africa in 1917 by Eduard Reichenow showed human-like *Plasmodium* parasites in the blood of captive chimpanzees and gorillas in Cameroon. Following Reichenow's observations, Blacklock and Adler in 1922 also described and confirmed *Plasmodium* parasites resembling *P. falciparum* in chimpanzees in Sierra Leone [25, 39, 40]. On the other hand, similar transmissions are also observed in the old and new-world monkeys. *P. cynomolgi* happens to be the first monkey *Plasmodium* species detected and characterised by Mayer in 1907 from a *Macaca cynomolgus* monkey [23, 41]. Further, observations by Robert Koch in Monkeys of East Africa in 1947, also served as the basis for discovering the third malaria cycle in primates [23, 28]. The work of Shortt and Garnham also further described malaria relapse or recrudescence in *P. cynomolgi* in 1948. Krotoski and co-workers also described the hypnozoite stages of the parasite [5, 23, 30, 42, 43].

5. Emerging zoonotic malaria and transmission concerns

Zoonotic malaria is an emerging form of malaria that affects and is shared by both humans and other mammals. Cross-species malaria transmissions have been observed with certain groups of *Plasmodium* species transmitted among different mammalian host species in nature and experimental settings. This raises concerns that borders on the need for one-health and it also indicates the possibility for susceptible mammals to double as reservoirs and hosts for their host-specific and non-specific *Plasmodium* species, which are competent enough to cause the disease across these mammal species. Secondly, frequent misdiagnosis of non-human *Plasmodium* species of malaria that infect humans is also a contributory factor. The continuous transmissions are also posited to have a great impact on human malaria eradication pegged for 2030 and the conservation of susceptible and highly endangered mammal species [31]. There are also knowledge gaps that are a source of concern and will require continuous and active research to ascertain the posited impact of this form of the disease. This will help develop effective mitigating actions to manage or deal entirely with such malaria transmissions.

Frequent passages of malaria parasite cell lines under laboratory conditions for certain lower mammal and vertebrate species have been successful. This has been adopted in the generation of human adaptable strains and mutants of *P. knowlesi*, *P. berghei*, *P. falciparum mutants 3D7 and Hb3* among others that are used for various malaria *in-vitro* studies [32, 37, 44–47]. The adaptability of such malaria parasite species to subsist and thrive on human red blood cells or non-human host red blood cells within cell cultures is an interesting observation to partly explain the multiple switch postulate, which is believed to account for the evolution of malaria parasites [48, 49]. This suggests that *Plasmodium* species has evolved with a high tendency to switch to different red blood cells among mammalian species. Though there are currently no known *Plasmodium* parasites of the lower mammalian species that infect humans in nature since culturing conditions are different from intact physiological conditions, however, it is envisaged that when given factors that frequently promote such contacts continue, human-adapted malaria parasite strains may evolve and circulate. Promoting factors such as laboratory spillovers, the presence of competent transmission vector, environmental conditions and host factors that bring proximity to the human-*Plasmodium* mutant interphase should be carefully investigated, and managed appropriately with this possibility in mind.

Non-human primate *Plasmodium* species are naturally and experimentally transmissible to humans and vice versa [31, 50–52]. Such cross-species infections are an emerging area of concern to current malaria transmission patterns facilitated by increased invasion, contact, and proximity to shared forest environments with non-human primates. Furthermore, host primates and vector confinement to certain geographic regions of the globe also influence the kind of circulating *Plasmodium* pathogen that can be transmitted [31, 35, 40]. Infections with *P. knowlesi* a type of monkey malaria, was the first zoonotic malaria to be described in 1965 to naturally infect humans [27–29, 39, 53]. Such infections are common within South East Asian countries where it is transmitted mainly by the vector *Anopheles balabacensis* [54]. *P. knowlesi* infections have been the main cause of malaria in Brunei and Singapore. In Malaysia, of the 2607 malaria cases reported in 2020, all were due to *P. knowlesi* infections with no report of any of the known human *Plasmodium* parasites. Malaria trends in Sabah over 5 years from 2014 to 2018 reveal that *P. knowlesi* over the period, accounted proportionally for 0.78 (13,569/17310) of all malaria cases which were reported [54].

Cases of fatal and mild forms of the disease due to *P. knowlesi* infections in humans have been reported in endemic communities, but the true prevalence is still not known [28, 55, 56]. Diagnosis using PCR aids in effective speciation and detection but the technique is not easily applicable in remote areas where the main host vertebrate *Macaca fascicularis* and human contacts are high. Methods such as microscopy are elusive due to their morphological resemblance to human *Plasmodium* parasites. Furthermore, whether current human infections are through the human-mosquito-human route or the Macaque-mosquito-human route, is not yet clear. Potential for natural human infections and experimental infection has also been demonstrated for other non-human primate *Plasmodium* species such as *P. cynomolgi*, *P. inui*, *P. brasilianum*, *P. coatneyi* and *P. simiovale* [57]. Putaporntip and coworkers after testing 1359 febrile human blood samples from 2007 to 2018 detected 9 cases of *P. cynomolgi* coinfections within 5 provinces in Thailand [58]. Further works by Yap and coworkers in 2021 also led to the detection of infections with *P. coatneyi (3)*, *P. cynomolgi (9)* and *P. inui (3)* among humans [59].

Apes are the main host of *Plasmodium* representatives of *Laverania* except for *P. falciparum,* which is a human *Plasmodium* pathogen [27, 60–62]. While Orangutans and Gibbons are found in Asia, Chimpanzees, Bonobos and Gorillas who are humans' closest relatives are found in Africa [39, 53, 60, 63, 64]. Such host and vector distribution patterns are important to note as they affect the disease transmission dynamics. Special *Plasmodium* species groups are known to uniquely infect the different Ape hosts of which most share a resemblance with the human *Plasmodium* versions. Besides these observations, *P. rodhain* and *P. schwetzi* infection in humans has been demonstrated and shown to be successful through blood inoculations [5, 23, 30, 62, 65]. Infections of Chimpanzees with *Plasmodium vivax* and *P. malariae* have also been demonstrated experimentally [60, 64, 66]. Another investigation into the prevalence of simian malaria identified *P. falciparum,* which was earlier thought to be a human-specific species for malaria infections to have naturally infected *Macaca radiata* and *Macaca mulatta* in India [51]. Suggesting that both humans and the great Apes could serve as reservoirs and hosts for human *Plasmodium* species and Ape *Plasmodium* parasite species. The consequence of reverse zoonosis is likely to evolve new and more virulent or attenuate existing species, which will likely change host and pathogen infection and transmission dynamics.

6. Path to the development of malaria

The establishment of the *Plasmodium* parasite in the blood of humans, non-human primates and other vertebrate hosts is important for malaria to occur [26, 67, 68]. This is mediated through a meal bite from a transmissible competent mosquito vector species harbouring infective stages of the parasite, this is important for malaria to occur as illustrated in **Figure 2** [69]. *Plasmodium* sporozoites after introduction into the host by the mosquito, invade hepatocytes and develop into merozoites, which further invade erythrocytes and develop into schizonts and gametocytes. For further perpetuation, gametocytes of *Plasmodium* are fed on by a mosquito and *Plasmodium* completes the sexual stages of their development to form asexual sporozoites and the cycle continues with another blood meal as illustrated below [69].

Clinical presentations of human malaria are well characterised and mainly known to be associated with cyclical fevers due to the continuous invasion, infection and re-infection of hepatocytes and erythrocytes by various stages of *Plasmodium* and the response reactions from the immune system of the host. In the uncomplicated scenario, the disease may be accompanied by chills, nausea, vomiting and headaches. Complicated malaria, which is a more severe form of the disease characterised by

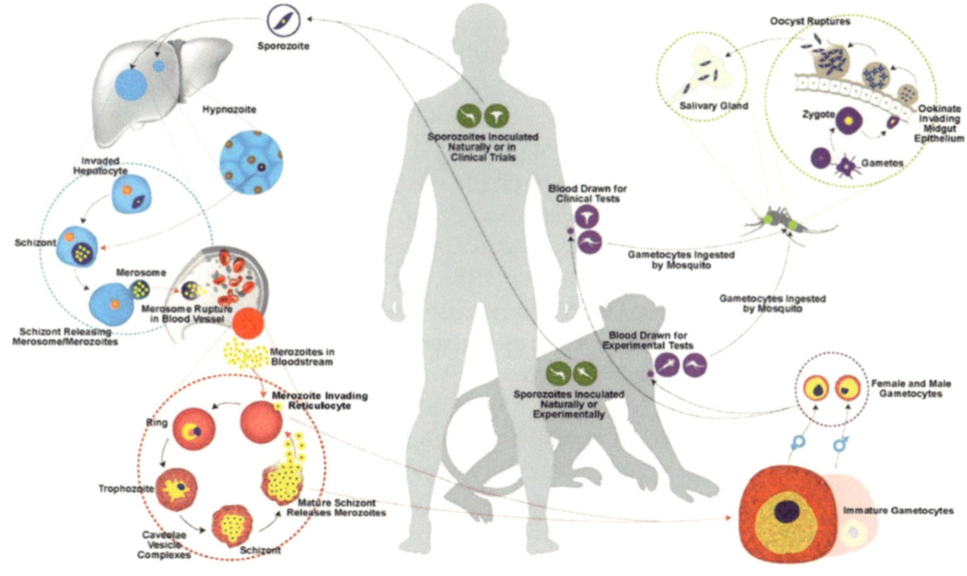

Figure 2.
Life cycle of Plasmodium *species involved in human and non-human primate transmissions [69].*

cerebral malaria with its accompanying seizures, severe malaria anaemia, coma, metabolic acidosis and death also, do occur. This is often seen among vulnerable groups such as children under 5 years of age, immune-compromised persons and persons with no pre-existing immunity. Furthermore, there is also malaria relapse caused by hypnozoites, which is associated with recurrent and difficult-to-treat malaria infections that may linger on for years.

6.1 Parasite development in vector

Mosquitoes become infected when they ingest human blood containing gametocytes. These gametocytes differentiate into male and female gametes within the mosquito's gut, facilitated by the mosquito's blood meal. Following fertilization, the zygote develops into a motile ookinete within 24 hours of having imbibed a blood meal. This extracellular ookinete then departs from the blood mass, navigates through the midgut epithelium and evolves into a growing oocyst in the basal subepithelial region located between the midgut epithelium and the basal lamina (BL) [70–72]. The midgut's peritrophic membrane (PM) functions as an initial defence line in *Anopheles* mosquitoes against ookinetes, providing a physical barrier [73]. Ookinetes release the chitinase enzyme to assist in navigating through the PM [74]. Similarly, ookinetes are confronted with midgut proteases. To counteract these proteases, ookinetes produce surface proteins called P25, P28 and P47, pivotal for their successful invasion of the midgut [75–77].

Several factors, such as the vector's type, parasite strain, environmental circumstances and host immunity, influence the development of the malaria parasite inside the vector. Vector competence refers to the inherent capacity of anopheline species or populations to facilitate the progression of *Plasmodium* parasites, transforming from ookinete to infective sporozoite [78]. Variation in vector competence occurs among different vectors and parasite combinations, and this variability can be influenced by genetic, molecular, immunological and ecological factors [78–81]. For instance, particular genes within mosquitoes can impact parasite infections, either amplifying or constraining their growth [81, 82]. Similarly, specific molecules produced by parasites can engage with the mosquito's immune system or midgut microbiota, enabling evasion or overcoming of the vector's defences [83, 84]. Additionally, environmental elements such as temperature, humidity, rainfall and seasonal variations can shape vector competence by influencing mosquito physiology, behaviour and lifespan [81, 84–86].

Managing malaria faces a significant challenge in light of the rise and spread of insecticide resistance within *Anopheles* mosquitoes. The emergence of resistance to insecticides can undermine the efficacy of strategies such as insecticide-treated nets (ITNs) and indoor residual spraying (IRS), which are designed to minimise human-mosquito interactions. While the precise mechanisms and outcomes are not entirely clear, insecticide resistance can also affect the abilities of malaria vectors, as indicated by a study [78]. Several studies have suggested that the impact of insecticide resistance on vector competence can fluctuate, depending on variables like the type of insecticide, the mechanism of resistance, the species of mosquito and the strain of the parasite. For instance, certain research has revealed that the rates of *Plasmodium* infection in pyrethroid-resistant mosquitoes can either increase or decrease compared to susceptible counterparts [78]. Furthermore, investigations have unveiled that insecticide resistance can have an impact on diverse facets of mosquito behaviour and fitness, including elements such as reproductive capacity, survival, feeding patterns and host preference. These factors, in turn, can shape the vectorial capacity, a measure of the potential for a mosquito population to transmit malaria [78]. As a result, it becomes crucial to observe and control insecticide resistance in malaria vectors, while simultaneously devising new methods and strategies to prevent or decrease the transmission of malaria.

6.2 *Plasmodium* parasites of malaria

Plasmodium species that cause malaria among vertebrates are diverse. The species responsible for causing malaria in humans are in five distinct forms: *Plasmodium falciparum*, *Plasmodium vivax*, *Plasmodium malariae*, *Plasmodium ovale sensu lato* (s.l.), which encompasses *P. o. curtisi and P. o. wallikeri* and *Plasmodium knowlesi* [55, 87]. Human *Plasmodium* species originate from different evolutionary lineages, sharing common ancestors with nonhuman primate species [25, 61, 88]. As anticipated, the five primary malaria-causing parasites exhibit distinct biological characteristics throughout their respective life cycles [5, 89].

One pivotal stage in this life cycle is the invasion of human red blood cells by *Plasmodium* species. While *P. falciparum* shows no particular preference for a specific age of red blood cells, *P. vivax* and the two species within *Plasmodium ovale sensu lato* (s.l.) tend to infect young red blood cells or reticulocytes. Conversely, *Plasmodium malariae* is thought to invade older red blood cells [90, 91]. Differences are also apparent in the timing and lifespan of gametocyte production, both of which are critical components of fitness [92, 93]. *Plasmodium falciparum* undergoes a more extended maturation process, spanning five stages over 9–12 days, and remains infectious for several days compared to other malaria parasites. In contrast, *Plasmodium vivax* and *P. ovale s.l.* have dormant stages or hypnozoites that lead to relapses after the initial infection; these stages are absent in *P. falciparum* and *P. malariae* [42, 94]. Another notable distinction is the ability of *P. falciparum*-infected red blood cells to adhere to the endothelium of capillaries and venules, a phenomenon called sequestration, which is associated with severe clinical symptoms uncommon in non-falciparum malaria [95, 96]. These traits represent only a fraction of the many variations among *Plasmodium* species causing malaria in humans.

In addition to *Plasmodium* species that primarily affect humans, there are zoonotic malaria parasites originating from nonhuman primates. The most prominent example is *Plasmodium knowlesi* found in macaques across Southeast Asia [55, 97–99]. However, evidence suggests that other nonhuman primate malaria species also function as zoonotic agents in this region, sometimes causing asymptomatic infections [99–101]. Moreover, anthropozoonotic malaria parasite cycles involving nonhuman primates in South America have been documented [41, 102, 103]. Despite the focus on zoonotic species, there are at least 39 known *Plasmodium* species affecting nonhuman primates globally, encompassing both formally described species and detected lineages [26, 67]. Some of these parasites received limited attention until recently, potentially due to challenges associated with studying nonhuman primates. Additionally, there was a significant emphasis on viable animal models to enhance the understanding of malaria biology and to explore treatment or vaccine options. Regardless of the factors that hindered their study, substantial progress has been made in the past two decades.

6.3 Biology and diversity of malaria vectors

Malaria is a severe and occasionally fatal illness caused by a parasite that infects specific mosquito species, which subsequently bite humans. The characteristics and variety of malaria carriers play a pivotal role in influencing malaria transmission and control. These carriers, belonging to the *Anopheles* genus, consist of over 400 species, with approximately 70 of them recognised as transmitters of malaria to humans [104]. Non-Primate transmissions are also facilitated by Mosquito vectors such as Aedes and Culex species.

The diversity of malaria vectors varies across different regions and habitats, contingent on environmental and climatic factors that impact their breeding, feeding and resting habits. Among the significant malaria carriers are *Anopheles gambiae sensu lato (s.l.), Anopheles funestus s.l., Anopheles arabiensis, Anopheles stephensi, Anopheles dirus, Anopheles minimus, Anopheles farauti, Anopheles darlingi* and *Anopheles albimanus* [104]. These vectors exhibit different preferences for host species, biting times, indoor or outdoor locations and larval habitats. For instance, *A. gambiae s.l.* is highly anthropophilic (prefers to feed on humans) and endophagic (feeds indoors), while *A. arabiensis* is more zoophilic (prefers to feed on animals) and exophagic (feeds outdoors) [105].

The genetic structure of malaria vectors' populations constitutes a pivotal facet of their biology and diversity, serving as a reflection of their evolutionary history, adaptability, gene flow and reproductive isolation. Population genetics aids in tracing the origin, distribution and movement of these vectors, as well as their susceptibility or resistance to insecticides and malaria parasites. Molecular methods like polymerase chain reaction (PCR), restriction fragment length polymorphism (RFLP), microsatellite analysis and DNA sequencing enable the assessment of genetic diversity and population structure of malaria vectors [106]. For example, PCR can distinguish the members of the *A. gambiae* complex, a group of morphologically similar sibling species differing in their vector capacities.

Comprehending the biology and diversity of malaria vectors is vital for grasping the epidemiology and ecology of malaria transmission, as well as for devising effective strategies for vector control. With knowledge about the attributes and behaviours of diverse malaria vectors in various settings, targeted interventions such as insecticide-treated nets (ITNs), indoor residual spraying (IRS), larval source management (LSM) and genetic modification (GM) can be employed [107]. However, the biology and diversity of malaria vectors are dynamic and influenced by factors like environmental shifts, human activities, insecticide resistance and parasite evolution. Consequently, ongoing monitoring and surveillance of malaria vectors remain indispensable for keeping information up to date and adapting interventions accordingly [107, 108].

7. Transgenic mosquitoes

Transgenic mosquitoes could be a successful choice for developing a range of effective disease-fighting strategies as a result of the advancements made in genetic modification in recent years [109–111]. Arthropod control by genetic modification is an old concept that was independently researched in the 1930s, 1940s and 1950s by three pioneers: A. S. Serebrovskii (1940), F. L. Vanderplank (1947) and E. F. Knipling (1955) [112, 113]. Furthermore, the 1970s saw a particular focus on studies concerning sterile males [109, 110, 114], which in turn prompted re-evaluation of the original concepts [109–111, 115–118].

The genetic modification of mosquitoes for the prevention of malaria is primarily focused on two main strategies: population suppression, which aims to eradicate or drastically reduce mosquito populations; and population modification, which aims to render the natural population immune to infection by expressing anti-plasmodial agents or altering mosquito genes crucial for parasite transmission [119–121]. Significant progress has been made in developing transgenic mosquitoes that are resistant to the parasites that cause malaria over the past 10 years. These developments include changes to mosquito genes essential for parasite development [122, 123] enhancement of mosquito immune components [124–126], the introduction of antiparasitic toxins or molecules [125, 127–129] and the expression of single-chain antibodies targeting parasite proteins [130, 131]. The creation of the first genetically modified mosquito in Africa through the Transmission Zero initiative holds special importance. This global scientific program is led by researchers from Imperial College London and the Ifakara Health Institute (IHI) in Tanzania, in collaboration with the Tanzanian National Institute of Medical Research (NIMR). This mosquito strain has been subject to genetic alterations that will ultimately provide researchers with the ability to hinder malaria transmission by mosquitoes. This noteworthy scientific achievement represents a pivotal advancement in the renewed worldwide efforts to eradicate malaria from the African continent [132].

The generation of transgenic mosquitoes poses a significant challenge, involving issues related to regulations, ethics and social aspects linked with the introduction of genetically modified organisms into the natural environment [133]. The transition of this approach from controlled laboratory settings to field trials in disease-endemic countries (DECs) is a gradual process aimed at maximising potential epidemiological benefits while minimising potential complications during implementation [134]. Among the multitude of factors to be taken into account is the irreversible nature of releasing organisms, as once released, it becomes exceedingly challenging to retrieve them in case issues emerge [133]. Unlike traditional methods of vector control, the utilisation of transgenic mosquitoes will encounter varying expectations from different stakeholders. Effective management of these divergent expectations is crucial to ensure ongoing support and mitigate opposition. This management is essential for a comprehensive assessment of potential public health benefits [134].

8. Environmental impact of *Plasmodium* transmission

Intriguingly the *Plasmodium* parasite sits on a knife edge as it will have to navigate different and mandatory environmental landscapes in a bid to survive and procreate. Traversing through the internal environment of a single or more than one vertebrate host or reservoir, the parasite is presented with a myriad of challenges including the need to usurp, manage or adapt to the varying degree of immunity presented by the host or reservoir as well as pressure from antimalarials if in use by the host. Moreover, co-infections be it with other *Plasmodium* species or other pathogens are also common and unique and may also influence susceptibility patterns of the host vertebrate to invasion and subsequently disease manifestation or an asymptomatic state. Host or reservoir interactions may be facilitated after entry of the pathogen via conduits such as a competent vector direct to the host, indirectly from the mother-to-child transmission and blood transfusion routes. The journey back to complete the sexual phase of the pathogen's development is precarious as it is greatly dependent on the survivability and existence of a competent vector. Vectoral characteristic consists of sex, feeding behaviour and time and state of internal and external parameters among others which are paramount to sustain the vector role to maintain the sexual stages of the *Plasmodium* parasite for further development and later transmission.

External environmental factors do influence the survival and the persistence of vectors and subsequently, enhance the transmission of their respective *Plasmodium* species. Factors promoting transmissions may include seasonal changes with a high prevalence of malaria cases and deaths linked to the wet season in most of Africa [107, 135, 136]. Mosquito populations and bites increase due to enabling conditions that facilitate the breeding of the vector throughout the wet period and summer [57, 105]. Another important factor is temperature, most of the vector species reduce their bites and also have their development from larvae to adult stage extended when temperatures are cold [57, 67, 105]. Changes in land use such as for Agriculture and irrigation, also provide breeding grounds for mosquitoes and a cool hiding place among growing plants for adult mosquitoes [137]. Invasion of the forest environment either legally for the construction of public goods like bridges and roads or illegally for hunting and exploitation of natural resources such as mining of minerals are on the increase, this exposes such workers to non-human primate mosquitoes [61, 137]. Uncovered created pools of water may serve as breeding grounds for mosquitoes. Fragmentation and indiscriminate or uncontrolled degradation of forests due to logging or the creation of human community settlements deplete forest tiers and also increase human exposure to non-human primate mosquitoes and *Plasmodium* species [137, 138].

Control and preventive programs for the external environment were designed to target mosquito vectors at all stages of development. Insecticide use, use of insecticide-treated bed nets, use of mosquito repellents, draining of swamps and puddles as well as wearing of protective garments that obscure the skin among others are used to exterminate mosquito populations or avoid their bites. Most of such earlier malaria control and elimination campaigns that adopted these strategies were not globally coordinated and though they made some achievements, they could not eliminate malaria or sustain the momentum. The use of chemicals such as DDT came along with its concomitant impact on human health and non-targeted fauna within the environment leading to disturbance in ecosystem balance and this has increased the dominance of some invasive species. The development of resistant mosquitoes to insecticides due to frequent usage has also been observed. Furthermore, DDT and organophosphate usage among other chemicals in Australia, have been shown to contribute to bird poisoning which is often characterized by birds falling from the skies [139]. This reveals the potential effect of DDT on humans through the food chain and other environmental conduits [139].

9. Ending malaria transmissions by 2030 the one-health way

Eradicating malaria by 2030 from the human population is achievable given the current strategies and coordinated momentum. The close observation of benchmarks and prompt interventions are robust. However, an entire win against malaria transmissions will demand a one-health approach to deal with possible re-invasion of *Plasmodium* and their respective vectors from animal reservoirs. This is a form of systems thinking that tackles at the same time, health matters with a human, animal and environmental outlook. Acting as a paradigm shift from the past approach of independent mono-health perspective adopted. Human health has always been the main agenda, ensuring a healthy environment will therefore demand a fair balance in already existing malaria control and elimination intervention programs. This will require the use of eco-health strategies involving environmental impact and risk assessment, which puts into perspective the consequence of interventions on the health of humans, animals, plants and other components of the environment. On one hand, there will be the need to improve surveillance of non-human primate malaria among non-human primates and humans. Enacting and enforcing conservation laws using strategies such as restoration, maintenance and regulation of deforestation will also be required to control the level of human invasions.

Mosquitoes are hematophagous and have been successful over many years serving as vectors for the transmission of malaria and other infectious diseases. The induction of selective pressures for the mosquito vector from transgenes or by-products of a poorly introduced control or preventive intervention may have dire consequences on malaria transmission and other mosquito-borne diseases [79, 123, 129, 140, 141]. Mosquito vectors under genetic pressures may select new preferences and competency for hosts, bridge and or transmit new infectious disease pathogens across the human-animal interphase. Healthy balance for ecosystems shared with mosquitoes during the introduction of vector control interventions will therefore be required at all times. It is the surest way to contribute to a sound and healthy world for all species involved. This will ensure that potential invasive organisms may not take the opportunity of the tilted balance to proliferate and eliminate other species from extinction. A well-coordinated research effort and shared data for humans, animals and the environment will be required. The recent transgenic mosquito trials ongoing in Tanzania are among the most wonderful achievements of the millennium with a promising outcome to contribute together with other adopted arsenals for eliminating malaria [124, 134]. This will require a careful evaluation of such programs with one health lens in order to be able to anticipate possible impacts on the environment and other species.

10. Conclusions

Fundamental to our understanding of malaria transmission today would have lingered on evasively for many years with its massive toll on human life except for the timely merger of past and current coordinated knowledge. Past information on malaria though was sparse and scattered; it still, resonates with the concept of one health which is a current paradigm for the achievement of holistic health. Drawing from careful observation of patient records, the unique cyclical nature of each *Plasmodium*-specific fever and environmental events associated with changes in seasonal patterns; land use, and hydrological distribution patterns. Though the level of knowledge in certain cases was not entirely accurate in the past, it paved the way for the discovery of medications for the disease, initiation and adoption of control and preventive interventions that caused a decline in malaria and are also very useful today. The corroborative involvement of the study of other vertebrate species was remarkable in unearthing some unsolved puzzles about the disease cycle and other aspects of malaria research. Zoonotic malaria is currently an emerging challenge and possibly ongoing within the African region where there are great Apes and also in South America. Drawing from the current widespread dominance of *P. knowlesi* malaria in Malaysia and some Southeast Asian countries, zoonotic malaria will require maximum attention to evaluate the changing dynamics in malaria transmission in these regions that bear the biggest burden of the disease. Past concentration skewed towards human-centred research and programs will require a one-health approach. These will include a well-coordinated approach involving human and animal programs, locale-specific friendly interventions and the environment at large to increase the tendency of achieving the malaria eradication target set for 2030 and beyond.

Conflict of interest

The authors declare no conflict of interest.

Author details

Jonas Bedford Danquah* and Jennifer Afua Afrifa Yamoah
Council for Scientific and Industrial Research, Animal Research Institute, Accra, Ghana

*Address all correspondence to: jonydan4@gmail.com

IntechOpen

© 2024 The Author(s). Licensee IntechOpen. This chapter is distributed under the terms of the Creative Commons Attribution License (http://creativecommons.org/licenses/by/3.0), which permits unrestricted use, distribution, and reproduction in any medium, provided the original work is properly cited.

References

[1] Carter R, Mendis KN. Evolutionary and historical aspects of the burden of malaria. Clinical Microbiology Reviews. 2002;**15**(4):564-594. DOI: 10.1128/CMR.15.4.564-594.2002

[2] Soren D. Can archaeologists excavate evidence of malaria?. World Archaeology: Archeology of Epidemics and Infectious Disease. 2003;**35**(2):193-209. DOI: 10.1080/0043824032000111371

[3] Soren D, Soren N. What killed the babies of Lugano. Archaeology. 1995;**48**(5):43-48

[4] Trájer AJ, Sebestyén V, Domokos E. The potential impacts of climate factors and malaria on the middle Palaeolithic population patterns of ancient humans. Quaternary International. 2020;**565**(October):94-108. DOI: 10.1016/j.quaint.2020.10.056

[5] Garnham PC. History of discoveries of malaria parasites and of their life cycles. History and Philosophy of Life Sciences. 1988;**10**(1):93-108

[6] Schats R. Developing an archaeology of malaria. A critical review of current approaches and a discussion on ways forward. International Journal of Paleopathology. 2023;**41**:32-42. DOI: 10.1016/j.ijpp.2023.03.002

[7] White NJ, Hien TT, Nosten FH. A brief history of Qinghaosu. Trends in Parasitology. 2015;**31**(12):607-610. DOI: 10.1016/j.pt.2015.10.010

[8] Unschuld PU, Tessenow H, Jinsheng Z. Huang Di Nei Jing Su Wen: Annotated Translation of Huang Di's Inner Classic – Basic Questions: 2 Volumes. California: University of California Press; 2011

[9] Boualam MA, Pradines B, Drancourt M, Barbieri R. Malaria in Europe: A historical perspective. Frontiers in Medicine. 2021;**8**(June):7-9. DOI: 10.3389/fmed.2021.691095

[10] Arrow KJ, Panosian C, Gelband H. Saving Lives, Buying Time: Economics of Malaria Drugs in an Age of Resistance. NW Washington D.C, United State of America: National Academies Press; 2004

[11] Cunha CB, Cunha BA. Brief history of the clinical diagnosis of malaria: From hippocrates to Osler. Journal of Vector Borne Diseases. 2008;**45**(3):194-199

[12] Retief F, Cilliers L. Malaria in Graeco-Roman Times. Acta Crystallographica. 2004;**47**(2004):127-137

[13] Kannadan A. History of the miasma theory of disease. ESSAI. 2018;**16**(18):41-43

[14] Neghina R, Iacobiciu I, Neghina AM, Marincu I. Malaria, a journey in time: In search of the lost myths and forgotten stories. The American Journal of the Medical Sciences. 2010;**340**(6):492-498. DOI: 10.1097/MAJ.0b013e3181e7fe6c

[15] Tizard IR, Musser JMB. Malaria and the ague. In: Great American Diseases their effects on the course of North American History. San Diego, CA United States of America: Academic Press; 2022. pp. 85-106

[16] Hume JCC, Lyons EJ, Day KP. Malaria in antiquity: Genetics perspective. World Archaeology. 2003;**35**(2):180-192. DOI: 10.1080/0043821000111362

[17] Jarcho S. Laveran's discovery in the retrospect of a century. Bulletin of the History of Medicine. 1984;**58**(2):215-224

[18] Capanna E. Grassi versus Ross: Who solved the riddle of malaria? International Microbiology. 2006;**9**(1):69-74

[19] Ross R. Sir Ronald Ross, 1857 to 1932. British Medical Journal. 1957;**1**(5033):1464-1466

[20] Hegner R. Sir Ronald Ross and the discovery of the mosquito transmission of malaria. The Journal of Parasitology. 1933;**19**(4):312-313

[21] WHO. Regional Data and Trends briefing kit: World Malaria Report 2022. Geneva – Switzerland; 2022

[22] Garnham PC. Distribution of simian malaria parasites in various hosts. The Journal of Parasitology. 1963;**49**(6):905-911

[23] Eyle DE. The species of simian malaria: Taxonomy, morphology, life cycle, and geographical distribution of the monkey species. The Journal of Parasitology. 1963;**49**(6):866-887

[24] Deichstetter P. The effect of climate change on mosquito-borne diseases. The American Biology Teacher. 2017;**79**(3):169-173

[25] Sharp PM, Plenderleith LJ, Hahn BH. Ape origins of human malaria. Annual Review of Microbiology. 2020;**74**:39-63. DOI: 10.1146/annurev-micro-020518-115628

[26] Faust C, Dobson AP. Primate malarias: Diversity, distribution and insights for zoonotic plasmodium. One Health. 2015;**1**:66-75. DOI: 10.1016/j.onehlt.2015.10.001

[27] Christophers R. Malaria from a zoological point of view. Proceedings of the Royal Society of Medicine. 1934;**27**(8):991-1000. DOI: 10.1177/003591573402700802

[28] Lee KS et al. *Plasmodium knowlesi*: Reservoir hosts and tracking the emergence in humans and macaques. PLoS Pathogens. 2011;**7**(4):e1002015. DOI: 10.1371/journal.ppat.1002015

[29] Cox-Singh J et al. *Plasmodium knowlesi* malaria in humans is widely distributed and potentially life threatening. Clinical Infectious Diseases. 2008;**46**(2):165-171. DOI: 10.1086/524888

[30] Collins WE, Skinner JC, Pappaioanou M, Broderson JR, Philip M. The Sporogonic cycle of *Plasmodium reichenowi*. The Journal of Parasitology. 2016;**72**(2):292-298

[31] Lempang MEP et al. Primate malaria: An emerging challenge of zoonotic malaria in Indonesia. One Health. 2022;**14**:100389. DOI: 10.1016/j.onehlt.2022.100389

[32] Carter R. On the genetics of malaria parasites, a memoir: Part I, rodent malaria parasites and the first genetic crosses. Parasitology International. 2022;**91**:102635. DOI: 10.1016/j.parint.2022.102635

[33] Chora ÂF, Mota MM, Prudêncio M. The reciprocal influence of the liver and blood stages of the malaria parasite's life cycle. International Journal for Parasitology. 2022;**52**(11):711-715. DOI: 10.1016/j.ijpara.2022.02.002

[34] Basco LK. Cultivation of asexual intraerythrocytic stages of *Plasmodium falciparum*. Pathogens. 2023;**12**(7):900. DOI: 10.3390/pathogens12070900

[35] Martinelli A, Culleton R. Non-human primate malaria parasites: Out of the forest and into the laboratory. Parasitology. 2018;**145**(1):41-54. DOI: 10.1017/S0031182016001335

[36] Sá MR. Studies of avian malaria and Brazil in the international scientific

context (1907-1945). História Ciencias, Saude - Manguinhos. 2011;**18**(2):499-518. DOI: 10.1590/s0104-59702011000200011

[37] Carter R. On the genetics of malaria parasites, a memoir: Part III, genetic crossing in human malaria parasites. Parasitology International. 2022;**91**:102639. DOI: 10.1016/j.parint.2022.102639

[38] Pattaradilokrat S, Wu J, Xu F, Su X. The origins, isolation, and biological characterization of rodent malaria parasites. Parasitology International. 2022;**91**:102636. DOI: 10.1016/j.parint.2022.102636

[39] Duval L, Ariey F. Ape Plasmodium parasites as a source of human outbreaks. Clinical Microbiology and Infection. 2012;**18**(6):528-532. DOI: 10.1111/j.1469-0691.2012.03825.x

[40] Duval L et al. African apes as reservoirs of *Plasmodium falciparum* and the origin and diversification of the Laverania subgenus. Proceedings of the National Academy of Sciences of the United States of America. 2010;**107**(23):10561-10566. DOI: 10.1073/pnas.1005435107

[41] Ta TH, Hisam S, Lanza M, Jiram AI, Ismail N, Rubio JM. First case of a naturally acquired human infection with *Plasmodium cynomolgi*. Malaria Journal. 2014;**13**(1):1-7. DOI: 10.1186/1475-2875-13-68

[42] Krotoski WA et al. Demonstration of hypnozoites in sporozoite-transmitted *Plasmodium vivax* infection. The American Journal of Tropical Medicine and Hygiene. 1982;**31**(6):1291-1293. DOI: 10.4269/ajtmh.1982.31.1291

[43] Shortt H. Saul Adler 1895 - 1966. Biographical Memoirs of Fellows of the Royal Society. 1967;**13**:1-34

[44] Basir R et al. *Plasmodium berghei ANKA* infection in ICR mice as a model of cerebral malaria. Iranian Journal of Parasitology. 2012;**7**(4):62-74

[45] Drew DR et al. Defining the antigenic diversity of *Plasmodium falciparum* apical membrane antigen 1 and the requirements for a multi-allele vaccine against malaria. PLoS One. 2012;**7**(12):e51023. DOI: 10.1371/journal.pone.0051023

[46] Jambou R, El-Assaad F, Combes V, Grau GE. In vitro culture of *Plasmodium berghei*-ANKA maintains infectivity of mouse erythrocytes inducing cerebral malaria. Malaria Journal. 2011;**10**:2-6. DOI: 10.1186/1475-2875-10-346

[47] Nkhoma SCet al. Dynamics of parasite growth in genetically diverse *Plasmodium falciparum* isolates. Molecular and Biochemical Parasitology. 2023;**254**(October 2022):111552. DOI: 10.1016/j.molbiopara.2023.111552

[48] Loy DE et al. Out of Africa: Origins and evolution of the human malaria parasites *Plasmodium falciparum* and *Plasmodium vivax*. International Journal for Parasitology. 2017;**47**(2-3):87-97. DOI: 10.1016/j.ijpara.2016.05.008

[49] Plenderleith LJ et al. Zoonotic origin of the human malaria parasite *Plasmodium malariae* from African apes. Nature Communications. 2022;**13**(1):1868. DOI: 10.1038/s41467-022-29306-4

[50] Voinson M, Nunn CL, Goldberg A. Primate malarias as a model for cross-species parasite transmission. eLife. 2022;**11**:1-27. DOI: 10.7554/eLife.69628

[51] Dixit J, Zachariah A, Sajesh PK, Chandramohan B, Shanmuganatham V, Karanth KP. Reinvestigating the status of malaria parasite (Plasmodium sp.) in Indian non-human primates. PLoS

Neglected Tropical Diseases. 2018;**12**(12):1-20. DOI: 10.1371/journal.pntd.0006801

[52] Prugnolle F, Rougeron V, Becquart P, Berry A, Makanga B, Rahola N. Diversity, host switching and evolution of *Plasmodium vivax* infecting African great apes. Proceedings of the National Academy of Sciences. 2013;**110**(20):8123-8128. DOI: 10.1073/pnas.1306004110

[53] Rayner JC, Liu W, Peeters M, Sharp PM, Hahn BH. A plethora of Plasmodium species in wild apes: A source of human infection? Trends in Parasitology. 2011;**27**(5):222-229. DOI: 10.1016/j.pt.2011.01.006

[54] Chua TH, Manin BO, Fornace K. Life table analysis of *Anopheles balabacensis*, the primary vector of *Plasmodium knowlesi* in Sabah, Malaysia. Parasites and Vectors. 2022;**15**(1):1-9. DOI: 10.1186/s13071-022-05552-9

[55] Antinori S, Galimberti L, Milazzo L, Corbellino M. *Plasmodium knowlesi*: The emerging zoonotic malaria parasite. Acta Tropica. 2013;**125**(2):191-201. DOI: 10.1016/j.actatropica.2012.10.008

[56] WHO. Expert Consultation on Plasmodium knowlesi Malaria to Guide Malaria Elimination Strategies, Kota Kinabalu, Malaysia, 1-2 March 2017: Meeting Report. Manila: WHO Regional Office for the Western Pacific. Switzerland; 2017

[57] Maeno Y et al. Humans frequently exposed to a range of non-human primate malaria parasite species through the bites of *Anopheles dirus* mosquitoes in south-central Vietnam. Parasites and Vectors. 2015;**8**(1):1-7. DOI: 10.1186/s13071-015-0995-y

[58] Putaporntip C, Kuamsab N, Pattanawong U. *Plasmodium cynomolgi* co-infections among symptomatic malaria patients, Thailand. Emerging Infectious Diseases. 2021;**27**(2):590-593

[59] Yap NJ et al. Natural human infections with *Plasmodium cynomolgi*, *P. inui*, and 4 other Simian Malaria Parasites, Malaysia. Emerging Infectious Diseases. 2021;**27**(8):2187-2191

[60] Boundenga L et al. Diversity of malaria parasites in great apes in Gabon. Malaria Journal. 2015;**14**(1):1-8. DOI: 10.1186/s12936-015-0622-6

[61] Pacheco MA, Cranfield M, Cameron K, Escalante AA. Malarial parasite diversity in chimpanzees: The value of comparative approaches to ascertain the evolution of *Plasmodium falciparum* antigens. Malaria Journal. 2013;**12**(1):1-20. DOI: 10.1186/1475-2875-12-328

[62] Escalante AA, Pacheco MA. Malaria molecular epidemiology: An evolutionary genetics perspective. Microbiology Spectrum. 2019;7(4):1-8. DOI: 10.1128/microbiolspec.ame-0010-2019

[63] De Nys HM, Löhrich T, Wu D, Calvignac-Spencer S, Hubertus Leendertz F. Wild African great apes as natural hosts of malaria parasites: Current knowledge and research perspectives. Primate Biology. 2017;**4**(1):47-59. DOI: 10.5194/pb-4-47-2017

[64] Prugnolle F et al. African great apes are natural hosts of multiple related malaria species, including *Plasmodium falciparum*. Proceedings of the National Academy of Sciences of the United States of America. 2010;**107**(4):1458-1463. DOI: 10.1073/pnas.0914440107

[65] Contacos PG, Coatney R. Experimental adaptation of simian malarias to abnormal hosts. The Journal of Parasitology. 1963;**49**(6):912-918

[66] Lefebvre MJM, Daron J, Legrand E, Fontaine MC, Rougeron V, Prugnolle F. Population genomic evidence of adaptive response during the invasion history of *Plasmodium falciparum* in the Americas. Molecular Biology and Evolution. 2023;**40**(5):1-16. DOI: 10.1093/molbev/msad082

[67] Chinh VD et al. Prevalence of human and non-human primate Plasmodium parasites in anopheline mosquitoes: A cross-sectional epidemiological study in Southern Vietnam. Tropical Medicine and Health. 2019;**47**(1):1-6. DOI: 10.1186/s41182-019-0139-8

[68] Joyner C et al. *Plasmodium cynomolgi* infections in rhesus macaques display clinical and parasitological features pertinent to modelling vivax malaria pathology and relapse infections. Malaria Journal. 2016;**15**(1):1-18. DOI: 10.1186/s12936-016-1480-6

[69] Galinski MR. Systems biology of malaria explored with nonhuman primates. Malaria Journal. 2022;**21**(1):1-38. DOI: 10.1186/s12936-022-04199-2

[70] Chandley P, Ranjan R, Kumar S, Rohatgi S. Host-parasite interactions during Plasmodium infection: Implications for immunotherapies. Frontiers in Immunology. 2023;**13**(January):1-27. DOI: 10.3389/fimmu.2022.1091961

[71] Gabrieli P et al. Mosquito trilogy: Microbiota, immunity and pathogens, and their implications for the control of disease transmission. Frontiers in Microbiology. 2021;**12**(April):1-17. DOI: 10.3389/fmicb.2021.630438

[72] Carter V, Nacer AML, Underhill A, Siden RE, Hurd H. Minimum ookinete to oocyst transformation in plasmodium. International Journal for Parasitology. 2007;**37**(March):1221-1232. DOI: 10.1016/j.ipara.2007.03.005

[73] Devenport M, Fujioka H, Donnelly-Doman M, Shen Z, Jacobs-Lorena M. Storage and secretion of Ag-Aper14, a novel peritrophic matrix protein, and Ag-Muc1 from the mosquito Anopheles gambiae. Cell and Tissue Research. 2005;**320**(1):175-185. DOI: 10.1007/s00441-004-1067-3

[74] Shahabuddin M, Kaslow DC. Plasmodium: Parasite chitinase and its role in malaria transmission. Experimental Parasitology. 1994;**79**:85-88

[75] Tomas AM et al. P25 and P28 proteins of the malaria ookinete surface have multiple and partially redundant functions. The EMBO Journal. 2001;**20**(15):3975-3983. DOI: 10.1093/emboj/20.15.3975

[76] Molina-Cruz A et al. The human malaria parasite Pfs47 gene mediates evasion of the mosquito immune system. Science. 2013;**340**(6135):984-987. DOI: 10.1126/science.1235264

[77] van Dijk MR et al. Three members of the 6-cys protein family of plasmodium play a role in gamete fertility. PLOS Pathogen. 2010;**6**(4):e1000853-e1000853. DOI: 10.1371/journal.ppat.1000853

[78] Suh PF et al. Impact of insecticide resistance on malaria vector competence: A literature review. Malaria Journal. 2023;**22**(1):1-11. DOI: 10.1186/s12936-023-04444-2

[79] Beerntsen BT, James AA, Christensen BM. Genetics of mosquito vector competence. Microbiology and Molecular Biology Reviews. 2000;**64**(1):115-137. DOI: 10.1128/mmbr.64.1.115-137.2000

[80] Tripet F, Aboagye-Antwi F, Hurd H. Ecological immunology of mosquito-malaria interactions. Trends

in Parasitology. 2008;**24**(5):219-227. DOI: 10.1016/j.pt.2008.02.008

[81] Lefevre T et al. Transmission traits of malaria parasites within the mosquito: Genetic variation, phenotypic plasticity, and consequences for control. Evolutionary Applications. 2018;**11**(4):456-469. DOI: 10.1111/eva.12571

[82] Huang W, Id SW, Id MJ. Self-limiting paratransgenesis. PLoS Neglected Tropical Diseases. 2020;**14**:1-9

[83] Dong Y, Manfredini F, Dimopoulos G. Implication of the mosquito midgut microbiota in the defense against malaria parasites. PLoS Pathogens. 2009;**5**(5):e1000423. DOI: 10.1371/journal.ppat.1000423

[84] Barletta ABF et al. Microbiota activates IMD pathway and limits Sindbis infection in Aedes aegypti. Parasites and Vectors. 2017;**10**(1):1-9. DOI: 10.1186/s13071-017-2040-9

[85] Kristan M, Abeku TA, Lines J. Effect of environmental variables and kdr resistance genotype on survival probability and infection rates in *Anopheles gambiae (s.s.)*. Parasites and Vectors. 2018;**11**(1):1-10. DOI: 10.1186/s13071-018-3150-8

[86] Field EN, Smith RC. Seasonality influences key physiological components contributing to *Culex pipiens* vector competence. Frontiers in Insect Science. 2023;**3**(May):1-9. DOI: 10.3389/finsc.2023.1144072

[87] Ansari HR et al. Genome-scale comparison of expanded gene families in *Plasmodium ovale wallikeri* and *Plasmodium ovale curtisi* with *Plasmodium malariae* and with other Plasmodium species. International Journal for Parasitology. 2016;**46**(11):685-696. DOI: 10.1016/j.ijpara.2016.05.009

[88] Escalante AA, Cepeda AS, Pacheco MA. Why *Plasmodium vivax* and *Plasmodium falciparum* are so different? A tale of two clades and their species diversities. Malaria Journal. 2022;**21**(1):1-19. DOI: 10.1186/s12936-022-04130-9

[89] Coatneyi GR, Collins WE, Warren M, Contacos PG. The Primate Malarias. Bethesda, Maryland, United State of America: Department of Health, Education and Welfare; 1971

[90] Kerlin DH, Gatton ML. Preferential invasion by *Plasmodium merozoites* and the self-regulation of parasite burden. PLoS One. 2013;**8**(2):1-9. DOI: 10.1371/journal.pone.0057434

[91] Gruszczyk J et al. Transferrin receptor 1 is a reticulocyte-specific receptor for *Plasmodium vivax*. Science. 2018;**359**(6371):48-55. DOI: 10.1126/science.aan1078

[92] Bousema T, Drakeley C. Epidemiology and infectivity of *Plasmodium falciparum* and *Plasmodium vivax* gametocytes in relation to malaria control and elimination. Clinical Microbiology Reviews. 2011;**24**(2):377-410. DOI: 10.1128/CMR.00051-10

[93] van de Vegte-Bolmer M et al. A portfolio of geographically distinct laboratory-adapted *Plasmodium falciparum* clones with consistent infection rates in anopheles mosquitoes. Malaria Journal. 2021;**20**(1):1-10. DOI: 10.1186/s12936-021-03912-x

[94] Robinson LJ et al. Strategies for understanding and reducing the *Plasmodium vivax* and *Plasmodium ovale* hypnozoite reservoir in Papua new Guinean children: A randomised placebo-controlled trial and mathematical model. PLoS Medicine. 2015;**12**(10):1-26. DOI: 10.1371/journal.pmed.1001891

[95] Bernabeu M et al. Severe adult malaria is associated with specific PfEMP1 adhesion types and high parasite biomass. Proceedings of the National Academy of Sciences of the United States of America. 2016;**113**(23):E3270-E3279. DOI: 10.1073/pnas.1524294113

[96] Brazier AJ, Avril M, Bernabeu M, Benjamin M, Smith JD. Pathogenicity determinants of the human malaria parasite *Plasmodium falciparum* have ancient origins. mSphere. 2017;**2**(1):1-13. DOI: 10.1128/msphere.00348-16

[97] Yusof R et al. Phylogeographic evidence for 2 genetically distinct zoonotic *Plasmodium knowlesi* parasites, Malaysia. Emerging Infectious Diseases. 2016;**22**(8):1371-1380. DOI: 10.3201/eid2208.151885

[98] Pramasivan S et al. Spatial distribution of *Plasmodium knowlesi* cases and their vectors in Johor, Malaysia: in light of human malaria elimination. Malaria Journal. 2021;**20**(1):1-12. DOI: 10.1186/s12936-021-03963-0

[99] Imwong M et al. Asymptomatic natural human infections with the simian malaria parasites *Plasmodium cynomolgi* and *Plasmodium knowlesi*. The Journal of Infectious Diseases. 2019;**219**(5):695-702. DOI: 10.1093/infdis/jiy519

[100] Raja TN et al. Naturally acquired human *Plasmodium cynomolgi* and *P. knowlesi* infections, Malaysian Borneo. Emerging Infectious Diseases. 2020;**26**(8):1801-1809. DOI: 10.3201/eid2608.200343

[101] Kotepui M, Masangkay FR, Kotepui KU, Milanez GDJ. Preliminary review on the prevalence, proportion, geographical distribution, and characteristics of naturally acquired *Plasmodium cynomolgi* infection in mosquitoes, macaques, and humans: A systematic review and meta-analysis. BMC Infectious Diseases. 2021;**21**(1):1-14. DOI: 10.1186/s12879-021-05941-y

[102] Lalremruata A et al. Natural infection of *Plasmodium brasilianum* in humans: Man and monkey share quartan malaria parasites in the Venezuelan Amazon. eBioMedicine. 2015;**2**(9):1186-1192. DOI: 10.1016/j.ebiom.2015.07.033

[103] De Oliveira TC et al. *Plasmodium simium*: Population genomics reveals the origin of a reverse zoonosis. The Journal of Infectious Diseases. 2021;**224**(11):1950-1961. DOI: 10.1093/infdis/jiab214

[104] Akuamoah-Boateng Y et al. Malaria transmission, vector diversity, and insecticide resistance at a peri-urban site in the forest zone of Ghana. Frontiers in Tropical Diseases. 2021;**2**(September):1-10. DOI: 10.3389/fitd.2021.739771

[105] Fondjo E et al. High vector diversity and malaria transmission dynamics in five sentinel sites in Cameroon. Malaria Journal. 2023;**22**(1):1-16. DOI: 10.1186/s12936-023-04552-z

[106] Weeraratne TC, Surendran SN, Walton C, Karunaratne SHPP. Genetic diversity and population structure of malaria vector mosquitoes *Anopheles subpictus*, *Anopheles peditaeniatus*, and *Anopheles vagus* in five districts of Sri Lanka. Malaria Journal. 2018;**17**(1):1-8. DOI: 10.1186/s12936-018-2419-x

[107] Koffi AA et al. Anopheles vector distribution and malaria transmission dynamics in Gbêkê region, central Côte d'Ivoire. Malaria Journal. 2023;**22**(1):1-12. DOI: 10.1186/s12936-023-04623-1

[108] Monroe A et al. Methods and indicators for measuring patterns of human exposure to malaria vectors.

Malaria Journal. 2020;**19**(1):1-14. DOI: 10.1186/s12936-020-03271-z

[109] Parres-Mercader M, Pance A, Gómez-Díaz E. Novel systems to study vector-pathogen interactions in malaria. Frontiers in Cellular and Infection Microbiology. 2023;**13**(May):1-13. DOI: 10.3389/fcimb.2023.1146030

[110] Su XZ, Zhang C, Joy DA. Host-Malaria parasite interactions and impacts on mutual evolution. Frontiers in Cellular and Infection Microbiology. 2020;**10**(October):1-20. DOI: 10.3389/fcimb.2020.587933

[111] Wyse AP, dos Santos AJB, Azevedo DJS, Meneses DAC, Santos VMDC. Mathematical modeling of the performance of wild and transgenic mosquitoes in malaria transmission. PLoS One. 2023;**18**(4 April):1-23. DOI: 10.1371/journal.pone.0285000

[112] Knipling EF. Possibilities of insect control or eradication through the use of sexually sterile males. Journal of Economic Entomology. 1955;**48**(4):459-462. DOI: 10.1093/jee/48.4.459

[113] Vanderplank FL. Experiments in the hybridisation of tsetse-flies (Glossin a, Diptera) and the possibility of a new method of control. Transactions of the Royal Entomological Society of London. 1947;**98**(1):1-18. DOI: 10.1111/j.1365-2311.1947.tb01049.x

[114] Curtis CF, Cook LM, Wood RJ. Selection for and against insecticide resistance and possible methods of inhibiting the evolution of resistance in mosquitoes. Ecological Entomology. 1978;**3**(4):273-287. DOI: 10.1111/j.1365-2311.1978.tb00928.x

[115] Bowman C, Gumel AB, Van Den Driessche P, Wu J, Zhu H. A mathematical model for assessing control strategies against West Nile virus. Bulletin of Mathematical Biology. 2005;**67**(5):1107-1133. DOI: 10.1016/j.bulm.2005.01.002

[116] Dyck VA, Hendrichs J, Robinson AS. Sterile Insect Technique: Principles and Practice in Area-Wide Integrated Pest Management. Dordrecht, The Netherlands: Springer Science & Business Media; 2005

[117] Amaku M, Coutinho FAB, Raimundo SM, Lopez LF, Nascimento Burattini M, Massad E. A comparative analysis of the relative efficacy of vector-control strategies against dengue fever. Bulletin of Mathematical Biology. 2014;**76**(3):697-717. DOI: 10.1007/s11538-014-9939-5

[118] Yao FA et al. Mark-release-recapture experiment in Burkina Faso demonstrates reduced fitness and dispersal of genetically-modified sterile malaria mosquitoes. Nature Communications. 2022;**13**(1):1-11. DOI: 10.1038/s41467-022-28419-0

[119] Pham TB et al. Experimental population modification of the malaria vector mosquito, *Anopheles stephensi*. PLoS Genetics. 2019;**15**(12):e1008440

[120] Adedeji EO et al. Anopheles metabolic proteins in malaria transmission, prevention and control: A review. Parasites and Vectors. 2020;**13**(1):1-30. DOI: 10.1186/s13071-020-04342-5

[121] Carballar-Lejarazú R et al. Next-generation gene drive for population modification of the malaria vector mosquito, *Anopheles gambiae*. Proceedings of the National Academy of Sciences of the United States of America. 2020;**117**(37):22805-22814. DOI: 10.1073/pnas.2010214117

[122] Corby-Harris V et al. Activation of akt signaling reduces the prevalence and intensity of malaria parasite infection and lifespan in Anopheles stephensi mosquitoes. PLoS Pathogens. 2010;**6**(7):1-10. DOI: 10.1371/journal.ppat.1001003

[123] Yamamoto DS, Sumitani M, Hatakeyama M, Matsuoka H. Malaria infectivity of xanthurenic acid-deficient anopheline mosquitoes produced by TALEN-mediated targeted mutagenesis. Transgenic Research. 2018;**27**(1):51-60. DOI: 10.1007/s11248-018-0057-2

[124] Dong S, Dong Y, Simões ML, Dimopoulos G. Mosquito transgenesis for malaria control. Trends in Parasitology. 2022;**38**(1):54-66. DOI: 10.1016/j.pt.2021.08.001

[125] Dong S, Fu X, Dong Y, Simões ML, Zhu J, Dimopoulos G. Broad spectrum immunomodulatory effects of *Anopheles gambiae* microRNAs and their use for transgenic suppression of Plasmodium. PLoS Pathogens. 2020;**16**(4):1-20. DOI: 10.1371/journal.ppat.1008453

[126] Dong Y, Das S, Cirimotich C, Souza-Neto JA, McLean KJ, Dimopoulos G. Engineered anopheles immunity to plasmodium infection. PLoS Pathogens. 2011;**7**(12):e1002458. DOI: 10.1371/journal.ppat.1002458

[127] Ito J, Ghosh A, Moreira LA, Wimmer EA, Jacobs-Lorena M. Acknowledgements competing interests statement transgenic anopheline mosquitoes impaired in transmission of a malaria parasite. Nature. 2002;**417**(May):452-455. [Online]. Available from: www.nature.com

[128] Moreira LA et al. Bee venom phospholipase inhibits malaria parasite development in transgenic mosquitoes. The Journal of Biological Chemistry. 2002;**277**(43):40839-40843. DOI: 10.1074/jbc.M206647200

[129] Yoshida S et al. Hemolytic C-type lectin CEL-III from sea cucumber expressed in transgenic mosquitoes impairs malaria parasite development. PLoS Pathogens. 2007;**3**(12):1962-1970. DOI: 10.1371/journal.ppat.0030192

[130] Isaacs AT et al. Transgenic *Anopheles stephensi* coexpressing single-chain antibodies resist *Plasmodium falciparum* development. Proceedings of the National Academy of Sciences of the United States of America. 2012;**109**(28):E1922-E1930. DOI: 10.1073/pnas.1207738109

[131] Isaacs AT et al. Engineered resistance to *Plasmodium falciparum* development in transgenic Anopheles stephensi. PLoS Pathogens. 2011;**7**(4):e1002017. DOI: 10.1371/journal.ppat.1002017

[132] Zero T. First Transgenic Mosquito Made in Africa by Transmission Zero. London, United Kingdom: Imperial College; 2023

[133] Huang W, Cha SJ, Jacobs-Lorena M. New weapons to fight malaria transmission: A historical view. Entomological Research. 2022;**52**(5):235-240. DOI: 10.1111/1748-5967.12585

[134] Knols BGJ, Bossin HC, Mukabana WR, Robinson AS. Transgenic mosquitoes and the fight against malaria: Managing technology push in a turbulent GMO world. American Journal of Tropical Medicine and Hygiene. 2007;**77**(SUPPL. 6):232-242

[135] Caminade C et al. Impact of climate change on global malaria distribution. Proceedings of the National Academy of Sciences of the United States of America. 2014;**111**(9):3286-3291. DOI: 10.1073/pnas.1302089111

[136] Rotimi K et al. Pharmacovigilance reporting during seasonal malaria chemoprevention campaign: Findings from Northern Nigeria. Scientific African. 2022;**17**:e01283. DOI: 10.1016/j.sciaf.2022.e01283

[137] van de Straat B et al. Zoonotic malaria transmission and land use change in Southeast Asia: What is known about the vectors. Malaria Journal. 2022;**21**(1):1-13. DOI: 10.1186/s12936-022-04129-2

[138] Multini LC, Wilke ABB, Marrelli MT. Neotropical anopheles (Kerteszia) mosquitoes associated with bromeliad-malaria transmission in a changing world. Acta Tropica. 2020;**205**:105413. DOI: 10.1016/j.actatropica.2020.105413

[139] Wildlife Health Australia. Pesticide toxicity in Australian native birds. WHA Fact sheet: Poisoning events in Australian wild birds. 2022. Available from: https://wildlifehealthaustralia.com.au

[140] Graboyes M, Meta J, Clarke R. Mazingira and the malady of malaria: Perceptions of malaria as an environmental disease in contemporary Zanzibar. Studies in History and Philosophy of Science. 2022;**95**:134-144. DOI: 10.1016/j.shpsa.2022.07.005

[141] Yamamoto DS, Sumitani M, Kasashima K, Sezutsu H, Matsuoka H. Inhibition of malaria infection in transgenic Anopheline mosquitoes lacking salivary gland cells. PLoS Pathogens. 2016;**12**(9):1-21. DOI: 10.1371/journal.ppat.1005872

Chapter 4

Malaria Transmission Dynamics in East Africa

Fred Anangwe Amimo

Abstract

Malaria remains one of the deadliest mosquito-borne diseases in the world and indeed in sub-Saharan Africa and the sub-region of East Africa. The sub-region ranges from the coastal landscapes of Kenya and mainland Tanzania to the east borders of the congolian tropical rain forest and river basin on west Uganda boundary. The many water bodies in the region provide breeding grounds for *Anopheles* mosquitoes which transmit malaria affecting large populations of humans. Domestic animals and wildlife also play a pivotal role in malaria transmission by providing micro-breeding and resting sites via their footprints and sheds. The dynamics of transmission of malaria therefore include the presence and behaviors of the *Anopheles* vectors, the prevalence of the *Plasmodium* parasites, seasonality, climate change and related environmental factors favoring transmission in East Africa, and affected human hosts. Rainfall patterns and temperature stand out in affecting both the vector and malaria parasite life cycle. Inadequate use of preventive measures and treatment regimens has increased the risk of transmission of the parasites. This chapter explores the dynamics and trends of malaria transmission in this part of Sub-Saharan Africa.

Keywords: malaria transmission, *Anopheles* mosquitoes, East Africa, *Plasmodium* parasites, dynamics

1. Introduction

Malaria is still one of the deadliest mosquito-borne diseases in the world and has remained the cause of many infections and deaths in East Africa [1, 2]. There are approximately 3500 known species of mosquitoes worldwide. Among them, the genus of *Anopheles* mosquitoes transmits malaria in sub-Saharan Africa. This genus contains more than 460 recognized species, and approximately 60–100 *Anopheles* species have been implicated in transmitting malaria parasites [2, 3]. East Africa is indeed a sub-region of Sub-Saharan Africa and is endowed with a tropical climate, diverse landscapes, and remarkable ecological features that are conducive for spread of malaria. The sub-region encompasses a large area, extending from the coastal areas of Kenya and mainland Tanzania to the western borders of Uganda and east Congo River basin. The Great Rift Valley, a geological trench that traverses these countries, is composed of escarpments, volcanoes, lakes, and hot springs and a unique tropical biodiversity within which *Anopheles* mosquitoes flourish and spread malaria.

At the core of East Africa is Lake Victoria whose basin supports year round malaria transmission. The lake provides important freshwater resources and sustains the livelihoods of millions of people who due to exposure to malaria have diverted their economic development in terms of these resources needed for prevention and cure of the disease [4]. Other lakes in the sub-region which experience malaria transmission include Lake Tanganyika, Lake Malawi, and the numerous freshwater lakes located in the Great Rift Valley. Malaria thrives in such areas with stagnant water, which serve as breeding grounds for mosquitoes. The presence of these lakes and other fresh water bodies in lowlands and some highland areas of East Africa have contributed to the prevalence of malaria. The *Anopheles* mosquitoes concurrently find suitable habitats for breeding within their bounds [5].

1.1 *Anopheles* breeding and proximity to human populations

Anopheles mosquitoes breed in relatively clean stagnant or slow-moving water bodies including water storage tanks, temporary pools, streams, river bank vegetation shelters, rice irrigation fields, ponds and swamps which are widespread in the sub-region [6]. In urban areas, *Anopheles* mosquitoes tend to breed in artificial water containers, such as jerricans, barrels, and discarded items that collect water. These breeding sites are often found in close proximity to human residences. Moreover, poorly maintained drainage systems and improper waste management have created stagnant water pools suitable for mosquito breeding in most of these urban areas. In rural areas *Anopheles* mosquitoes breed in natural water bodies like streams, river banks, ponds, and swamps. These breeding sites are often located in close proximity to human settlements, particularly in areas where water sources are shared between the inhabitants and breeding by mosquitoes [7]. A case in point is the village communities living in vicinity of rivers and areas with rice irrigation fields in which the paddies provide breeding grounds for *Anopheles* mosquitoes. The many rice irrigation schemes in the sub-region have attracted huge settlements where immune and non-immune human populations provide labor in the fields and thereby come into close proximity of breeding sites of the *Anopheles* vectors of malaria.

Common human behaviors in East Africa such as storing water in containers or engaging in outdoor activities near water bodies creates additional breeding sites for mosquitoes unintentionally. Furthermore, settlement patterns in this region show a pattern of close proximity of houses to water bodies, which affects the distance between breeding sites and human populations. However, the specific distance between *Anopheles* mosquito breeding habitats and human populations differ widely and are determined by local environmental and socio-economic factors. The traditional east African type of house constructed in lowlands is mosquito permissive and contributes to massive entry of *Anopheles* mosquitoes into the houses mainly through the eyes and bite inhabitants without treated bed nets thereby increasing the chances of malaria infection.

1.2 Role of domestic animals

While humans are the primary hosts for malaria parasites, mosquitoes feed on both humans and animals, and some domestic animals have been found to contribute to the dynamics of malaria transmission in the region. Female *Anopheles* mosquitoes require blood meals to complete their reproductive cycle. Besides feeding on humans, they bite and feed on domestic animals, including cattle, goats, sheep, pigs and dogs.

Domestic animals have indeed been implicated in influencing the abundance and density of *Anopheles* mosquitoes. Livestock, such as cattle and goats, provide blood meals for mosquitoes, which support their survival and reproduction. Areas of East Africa with higher livestock populations tend to experience increased mosquito densities, which subsequently elevate the risk of malaria transmission to both humans and animals [8]. Cattle require water for drinking, and their presence near water bodies have contributed to the creation of additional breeding habitats for *Anopheles* mosquitoes. Cattle troughs, footprints, watering holes, and areas where animals congregate providing suitable breeding sites for mosquitoes when the water becomes stagnant or poorly drained.

1.3 Vegetation cover

Vegetation, inclusive of forests, savannas, dense vegetation near water bodies, and maize plantations provide suitable breeding sites for *Anopheles* mosquitoes. These vegetation areas usually have natural depressions, puddles, whorled leaves or small pools of water that collect rainwater, creating stagnant water bodies where mosquitoes lay their eggs. High vegetation coverage near human settlements increases the likelihood of mosquito breeding sites in close proximity to human populations. Changes in vegetation coverage due to deforestation, land conversion for agriculture, and urbanization has contributed to mosquito breeding and malaria transmission. Deforestation, for example, has led to alterations in mosquito habitat availability, water availability, and human-animal interactions, potentially influencing the transmission of the disease [9]. The dynamics of the role of vegetation cover in *Anopheles* mosquito breeding depend on factors such as the prevalence of mosquito vector species, change in temperatures and variable rainfall patterns in the local habitats.

2. Components of malaria transmission dynamics

East Africa is known to have a high burden of malaria attributable to *Anopheles* mosquito vectors with several factors contributing to its transmission [10]. Malaria transmission dynamics in the sub-region is therefore characterized by the presence of the *Anopheles* mosquito vector species, the *Plasmodium* parasites that cause the disease, human host factors, and environmental factors including transmission seasonality and climate change [11].

2.1 *Anopheles* species and *Plasmodium* parasites

The primary mosquito vectors responsible for malaria transmission in East Africa are mainly *Anopheles gambiae*, *An. arabiensis* and *An. funestus*. These mosquito species thrive in the region's diverse ecological backgrounds, including urban centers and rural areas of both lowland and highland settings. In Kenya, mainland Tanzania, and Uganda *An. gambiae and An. funestus* are the most efficient and widespread mosquito vectors. They breed in various water bodies, such as stagnant puddles, rice fields, irrigation channels, and river edges [11–13]. The most prevalent species of malaria parasites in the sub-region are *Plasmodium falciparum*, which is responsible for severe cases and most malaria-related deaths, and *Plasmodium vivax*, which is less common but still present in some areas. *Plasmodium falciparum* is the most deadly of all malaria parasites and is responsible for the majority of severe malaria cases and malaria-related deaths in East Africa [14]. It is known for its ability to rapidly multiply in the bloodstream and cause severe complications, such as cerebral malaria and severe anemia. *Plasmodium vivax* has the unique ability to form dormant liver stages, the hypnozoites, which can lead to recurrent infections even after successful treatment of the acute phase [15] thus propagating transmission further.

2.2 Human host factors

The risk of malaria infection is influenced by various human factors. These include individual immune responses, genetic factors, previous exposure to malaria, their behavior, nutritional status and travel among others. Vulnerable community members pertaining to severe malaria include young children, pregnant women, non-immune individuals and those with weakened immunity probably from malnutrition common in the region. With acquired immunity, those in the region living in endemic areas have developed partial immunity over time through constant repeated exposure to *Plasmodium* parasites. Among those living in endemic regions such as around Lake Victoria are cases of genetic variants of sickle cell trait that are less vulnerable to malaria infection. Behaviorally, there is a tendency for some people who live in areas with high mosquito density and have not embraced usage of repellents and mosquito nets risking being bitten by infected mosquitoes. With much poorly constructed homes and limited access to health facilities for diagnosis and treatment, malaria has remained a significant public health challenge in East Africa, leading to substantial morbidity and mortality, particularly among pregnant women and children under 5 years of age [12].

2.3 Transmission seasons and suitable conditions

East Africa's diverse landscapes, from coastal regions to high-altitude areas, play a significant role in malaria transmission. Mosquito breeding sites, such as stagnant water bodies, are abundant, and suitable climatic conditions support the survival and reproduction of both mosquitoes and parasites. Kenya's diverse climate, characterized by distinct wet and dry seasons, significantly influences malaria transmission patterns. In all other major East African Countries, there is an increase in mosquito breeding sites due to the accumulation of water during the rainy season. The high humidity and temperatures during this period accelerate mosquito development and the incubation of malaria parasites within the mosquitoes [16–18]. Malaria transmission in the region is seasonal, with peak transmission occurring during and after the rainy seasons when mosquito breeding sites increase. This seasonality leads to fluctuations in malaria incidence, with higher transmission rates during the wetter months. The availability of suitable breeding sites, especially during the rainy season, facilitates the rapid proliferation of these mosquito populations, leading to increased malaria transmission.

3. Underlying factors in malaria transmission

3.1 Malaria vector presence

In East Africa, several *Anopheles* mosquito species are known to be important vectors of malaria. The predominant species vary in different regions and over time due to various factors, including environmental conditions and human interventions.

Precisely, the *Anopheles* mosquito species commonly associated with malaria transmission in East Africa are *Anopheles gambiae* complex and *Anopheles funestus*. The *Anopheles gambiae* complex contains multiple sibling species, including *Anopheles gambiae* and *Anopheles arabiensis* [19]. *Anopheles gambiae* is often the most important malaria vector in many parts of East Africa, while *Anopheles arabiensis* is also a significant contributor to malaria transmission. *Anopheles funestus* is found in various parts of East Africa and also plays a significant role in malaria transmission. The relative abundance and distribution of these species varies across different areas of the sub-region and may also change over time.

3.2 Distribution and density of *Anopheles* mosquitoes

The distribution of the various *Anopheles* mosquito species which are associated with malaria transmission in East African countries of Kenya, mainland Tanzania and Uganda include *Anopheles gambiae*, which is widespread in sub-Saharan Africa. Other countries in sub-Saharan Africa where *An. gambiae* is found are Nigeria, Ghana, Burkina Faso, Cameroon, and Sudan among others. *Anopheles funestus* is found in widespread areas of East Africa and extends further south in countries such as Mozambique, Malawi, Zambia, Zimbabwe, and parts of South Africa. *Anopheles arabiensis* is prevalent in sub-Saharan Africa, and includes Kenya and mainland Tanzania among others such as Ethiopia, Sudan, and Somalia. It is particularly known for its adaptability to arid and semi-arid environments. *Anopheles merus* is primarily found in coastal areas of East Africa, including parts of Kenya and mainland Tanzania. *Anopheles coustani* is not only found in East Africa but also parts of West and Central Africa. *Anopheles rivulorum,* a closely related species to *Anopheles funestus* is found in various parts of Africa, including East and West Africa. A new entrant species, *Anopheles stephensi* has recently invaded East Africa but is originally predominantly found in parts of Asia, including countries such as India, Pakistan, Iran, Iraq, Afghanistan, and Saudi Arabia [19]. These malaria mosquitoes exhibit some degree of geographic variation within their ranges and their distribution may not be limited to the countries mentioned above, as they may be present in neighboring regions.

Malaria transmission by *Anopheles* mosquito species in East Africa vary in density [20–22]. *An. gambiae* is often the most important vector in many parts of East Africa. It typically prefers breeding in sunlit water bodies such as small temporary pools, puddles, and agricultural fields. It is adapted to both rural and urban environments and exhibits a preference for biting humans. *Anopheles funestus* is another major malaria vector in East Africa, particularly in areas with higher rainfall and more permanent water bodies. It commonly breeds in large, permanent bodies of water like swamps, lakes, and rivers. It is typically more active during the early evening and late night hours, and it tends to bite both humans and animals. *Anopheles arabiensis* is known for its ability to adapt to various ecological settings. It exhibits a preference for breeding in temporary water bodies, including small rain pools, agricultural fields, and human-made containers. It is commonly found in rural areas and is often active during the early evening and early morning hours. *Anopheles merus* overall contribution to malaria transmission may vary depending on local conditions and its relative abundance compared to other species. *Anopheles coustani* plays a lesser role in malaria transmission compared to species like *An. gambiae* s.s. and *An. funestus*. It is more commonly found in savannah and grassland regions and exhibits a preference for biting both humans and animals [14].

3.3 Areas of high transmission of *Plasmodium* parasites

As depicted in **Figure 1** the areas of high transmission for *Anopheles* mosquito species vary within East Africa depending on factors such as climate, geography, and local ecological conditions [24]. The precise distribution and intensity of malaria transmission may vary within these regions, influenced by factors such as climate variations, human population movements, and the prevalence of malaria parasites [14]. Warmer temperatures shorten the development time of the *Plasmodium* parasites within the mosquito, leading to increased transmission rates. Changes in rainfall patterns experienced in parts of East Africa are responsible for creation of breeding sites for mosquitoes, affecting their abundance. The high population movements including travel in East Africa, has introduced malaria infected individuals to new areas triggering outbreaks of malaria especially in highlands where many susceptible individuals live.

The Entomological Inoculation Rate (EIR) referring to the number of infectious mosquito bites received by an individual per year is a crucial epidemiological measure used to assess the intensity of transmission of malaria. The EIR is higher in areas with high mosquito density, favorable breeding conditions, and high malaria prevalence in humans compared to areas with lower malaria prevalence [24, 25]. *Anopheles gambiae* is known to be highly efficient in transmitting malaria parasites, particularly *Plasmodium falciparum*, which remains the most common in the region and highly virulent. The EIR has been used in East Africa to gauge the risk of malaria infection faced by local populations. Surveys involving human landing catches and indoor mosquito trapping have been carried out to estimate mosquito biting rates and the proportions of mosquitoes infected with *Plasmodium* parasites [22, 26].

3.4 Prevalence and diversity of *Plasmodium* species

Malaria, caused by *Plasmodium* parasites, is a major public health concern in East Africa. The region is highly endemic for malaria, with transmission occurring throughout the year, although intensity may vary across different areas and seasons. The main species of *Plasmodium* responsible for malaria in East Africa is *Plasmodium falciparum*, which is the most virulent species and responsible for the majority of malaria-related deaths, and *Plasmodium vivax*, which is less prevalent but can cause relapses of the disease [24]. High parasite prevalence is bound to increase the chances of the *Anopheles* mosquitoes acquiring infection from human hosts during blood feeding and eventually transmitting it to other persons [27]. The prevalence of *Plasmodium* parasites in East Africa is influenced by several factors, including climate, geography, human behavior, and socioeconomic conditions. Malaria transmission is facilitated by the presence of competent mosquito vectors, primarily *Anopheles* mosquitoes, which breed in various types of water bodies, such as stagnant pools, swamps, and rice fields. The high humidity and temperature in many parts of East Africa provide favorable conditions for mosquito breeding and parasite development [28].

3.5 Seasonality, altitude and related factors

Seasonality, altitude, and other related factors play significant roles in malaria occurrence and transmission in East Africa [24]. Malaria transmission in East Africa often exhibits seasonal patterns, with higher transmission rates during certain times of the year. The exact timing and duration of the peak transmission season varies

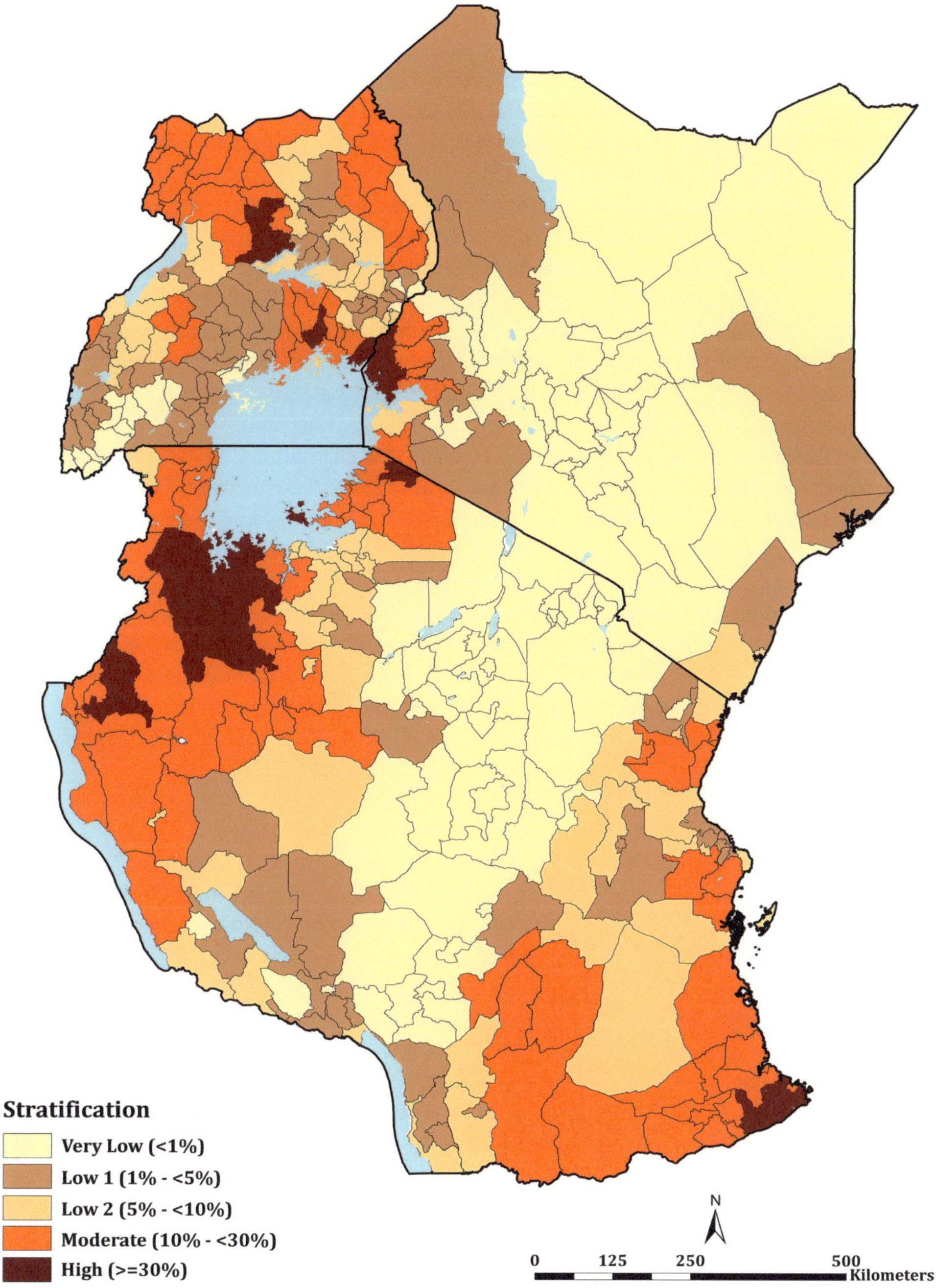

Figure 1.
Plasmodium falciparum *parasite prevalence in East Africa [23].*

across different regions and countries. Generally, the transmission increases during or after the rainy season when there is an abundance of mosquito breeding sites. The rainy season provides optimal conditions for mosquito reproduction and survival, leading to increased malaria transmission. However, in some areas with irrigation schemes or areas with perennial transmission, malaria may occur throughout the year [13, 29]. Altitude has a significant impact on malaria transmission in East Africa. Generally, malaria transmission decreases as altitude increases. This is because the *Anopheles* mosquitoes, which are the primary vectors for malaria, have specific altitude preferences. These mosquitoes thrive in low-lying areas and are less common at higher altitudes due to the cooler temperatures and less favorable environmental conditions. Therefore, highland areas in East Africa, particularly those above 2000 meters, tend to have lower malaria transmission rates compared to lowland areas.

Several other factors influence malaria occurrence and transmission in East Africa, including vector species, climate change and socioeconomic factors. The presence and abundance of specific mosquito vector species may affect the transmission dynamics. Different *Anopheles* mosquito species have varying preferences for breeding sites, feeding behavior, and susceptibility to *Plasmodium* parasites. Human activities, such as agricultural practices, deforestation, and settlement patterns, have an impact on malaria transmission. Changes in land use and water management practices may create or modify mosquito breeding sites, increasing the risk of malaria transmission. Climate variability and change may influence malaria transmission patterns in East Africa. Changes in temperature, rainfall patterns, and humidity levels may impact mosquito breeding, parasite development, and the geographic distribution of both the vectors and the parasites [30, 31]. Poverty, limited access to healthcare services, and inadequate infrastructure may contribute to the persistence and burden of malaria. These factors may affect the availability and utilization of preventive measures, diagnosis, and treatment options, leading to higher malaria transmission rates [25]. The specific influence of these factors may vary within different countries and regions of East Africa.

4. Malaria transmission trends

Figure 2 depicts general trends of malaria transmission in East Africa. The transmission in the region is a complex interplay of various factors, including an enabling environment and habitats for breeding consisting of suitable water bodies, landscapes, vegetation, altitude and the phenomena of climate change. The conducive breeding environment yields three efficient vectors of malaria: *Anopheles gambiae*, *An. funestus,* and *An. arabiensis* among others. Due to their efficiency, female *Anopheles* mosquitoes infected with *Plasmodium* parasites from a previous human blood meal develop a tight relationship in which the parasites undergo sexual reproduction, fertilization and develop from zygote into ookenetes in the midgut and migrate to the body cavity as oocysts which multiply and rupture to release sporozoites. The sporozoites migrate to the salivary glands. At the next available blood meal, the mosquito vectors pass on the infective sporozoites into a new human hosts' blood and into the liver in form of merozoites. Merozoite introduction into the bloodstream causes malaria. Both human and domestic animal hosts interact with the environment in a delicate balance where if not treated, newly emerged adult females acquire parasites afresh from infected individuals and the transmission continues unabated.

In order to determine the level of infection in relation to transmission of malaria in East Africa, various methods and data sources may be employed to provide data on prevalence rates, transmission intensity, and intervention efforts in the region. Existing data sources and detailed reports on malaria transmission are available with organizations such as World Health Organization (WHO), Centers for Disease Control Malaria Information and the Malaria Atlas Project (MAP) [32–34]. The Lake Basins and the coastal regions in East Africa are endemic for malaria. These regions

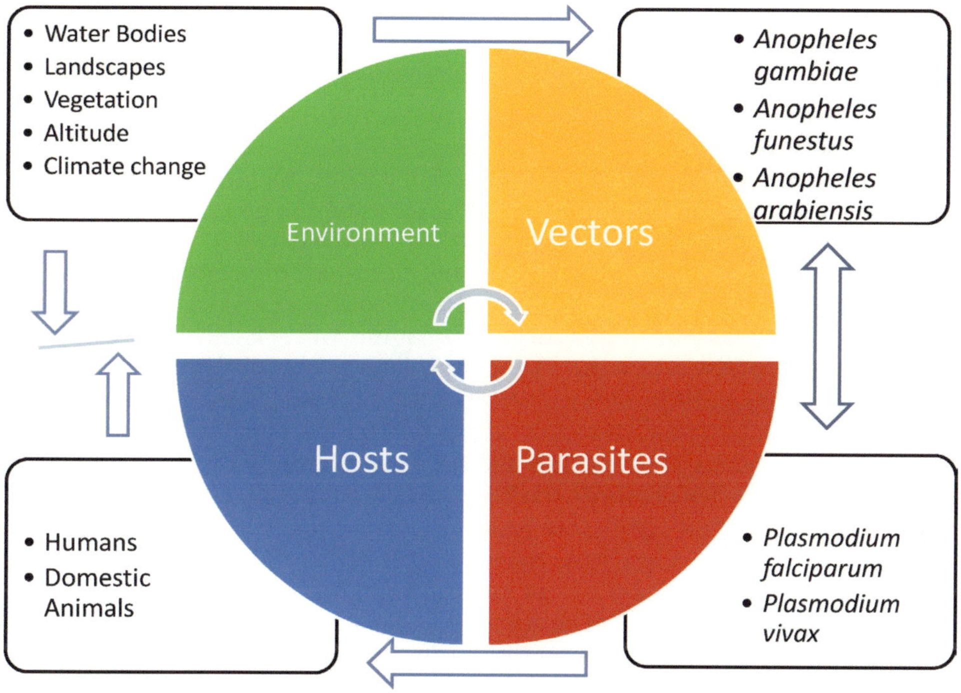

Figure 2.
Malaria transmission in East Africa (by author).

experience higher transmission rates of malaria attributed to the climate and vector abundance. To provide insights into reported malaria cases from local health facilities and determine trends and prevalence rates of malaria, analysis of epidemiological data from surveillance systems is procedural contributing to determination of the level of infection. Alongside, vector surveillance is often conducted to assess vector abundance and *Anopheles* distribution in the region. Monitoring *Anopheles* presence and behavior is crucial for understanding transmission patterns [35–37].

Blood sampling and laboratory analysis is carried out in local laboratories to measure *Plasmodium* parasite prevalence and to determine the prevalence of malaria parasites among human populations in the region through conducting surveys in affected areas [38]. Interventions such as Long Lasting Insecticide Nets (LLINs), Indoor Residual Sprays (IRS) and administration of malaria drugs are assessed to help determine the existing level of transmission and gauge their impact [39]. Collaboration between researchers and local health authorities is crucial in providing and updating data on insights on the overall levels of infection [27].

5. Role of interventions and challenges

Interventions have mainly aimed at controlling *Anopheles* mosquitoes using (LLINs) and IRSs, preventing the spread of *Plasmodium* parasites, and reducing incidence of the disease through improved access to diagnostics and treatment. Long-lasting Insecticide Nets have proved effective at protecting individuals during sleep while IRS has targeted high transmission areas where *Anopheles* mosquito densities are high. These interventions are proving successful in some areas of East Africa, but there are challenges and limitations experienced regionally that lead to their limitation in impacting reduction in malaria transmission.

5.1 Transmission persistence

Emergence of insecticide-resistant *Anopheles* mosquito populations is widespread in the region attributed to pyrethroids used in LLINs and IRS programs. This has led to interventions becoming less effective in controlling the mosquito populations and gradually malaria transmission has persisted in areas where insecticide resistance is prevalent [26, 40, 41]. The malaria parasites have also developed resistance to treatment by some anti-malarial drugs such as chloroquine, which hampers the effectiveness of treatment interventions and further translates into persistence of malaria in the local population. High transmission of malaria is evident in some remote and impoverished areas of East Africa where access to healthcare facilities for treatment is lacking and people are often not diagonized and prescribed appropriate antimalarial drugs. Delayed or inadequate treatment has contributed to resistant forms of malaria and persistence of transmission in the region.

The East African Community has embraced population movement for economic enhancement; however, this movement has contributed to the spread of malaria into new horizons or into areas where the disease had been controlled. Such movement and other behavioral tendencies including outdoor activities during peak mosquito biting hours of evening and early in the morning expose people and increase the risk of mosquito bites and subsequent malaria infection. In some cases misconceptions about malaria prevention and treatment contributes to delays in seeking appropriate healthcare, aggravating transmission [42]. Lack of community acceptance of an intervention due to local beliefs has hampered success of some interventions. For instance, inconsistent use of bed nets and failure to adhere to treatment regimens reduces the impact of these interventions and provides for further transmission. Factors such as socio-economic status, education, cultural superstitions and practices influence the uptake of these interventions [43].

5.2 Changes in climate

Changes in climate have influenced mosquito breeding patterns and spread of malaria. Climate change has resulted in the expansion of geographical ranges of *Anopheles* mosquito vector populations and *Plasmodium* parasites, contributing to persistent transmission. Climate Variability has affected mosquito breeding habitats and influenced the distribution and abundance of *Anopheles* mosquitoes. Changes in temperature and rainfall patterns create new opportunities for mosquito breeding and alter the timing of peak transmission seasons [44]. Temperature affects both the *Anopheles* mosquito and *Plasmodium*'s life cycle in the vector. The daily temperature variation influences the survival, development, and reproduction rates of mosquitoes. Stagnant water after increased rainfall provides ideal conditions for mosquito larvae to thrive. Humid conditions and elevated temperatures in the region result into faster development rates for the mosquito from egg to adult, which translates into more rapid population growth. Due to the foregoing climatic changes the extrinsic incubation period, which is the time required for *Plasmodium* parasites to complete development within the malaria mosquito before transmission to a new host, is shortened thereby perpetuating transmission.

5.3 Vector behavior and outdoor transmission

In areas of high bed net coverage, *Anopheles* mosquitoes in East Africa have exhibited changes in their feeding behavior, with an increasing proportion of bites occurring outdoors and at times when people are not protected by bed nets [45]. This behavioral resistance reduces the effectiveness of indoor-based interventions leading to residual malaria transmission. Research and surveillance efforts have been hampered in the absence of understanding the behavior of outdoor biting mosquitoes. Outdoor resting sites for *Anopheles* mosquitoes have created alternative breeding and resting sites, a pattern that continues to contribute to transmission in the absence of wearing protective clothing and using repellents, especially during times when bed nets may offer limited protection.

5.4 Sub-optimal implementation of integrated strategies

Lack of integration of interventions hinders their effectiveness when they are implemented in isolation [46]. A case in point in the region is when vector control measures in some areas are not accompanied with case management propagating transmission rates due to untreated cases alongside concurrent mosquito breeding. Limited impact on transmission is also evident when mosquito behavior, human behavior and changes in environmental conditions are not addressed in combination leading to suboptimal results. The risk of resurgence in cases of malaria is imminent in the region without a comprehensive approach in implementing interventions. Focus on one intervention is the cause of emergence of resistant *Anopheles* mosquitoes and *Plasmodium* parasites in some areas of East Africa which continues to reduce the long-term effectiveness of interventions [47].

6. Conclusion

Malaria, a life-threatening mosquito-borne disease caused by *Plasmodium* parasites, continues to be a major public health concern in East Africa. The region, comprising of the countries Kenya, mainland Tanzania, and Uganda, is characterized by ecological features, a typical tropical climate and landscape endowed with the Great Rift Valley, lakes and lake basins which contribute to creation of breeding habitats for *Anopheles* mosquitoes. Most of these areas are relatively close to human dwellings. The proximity of *Anopheles* mosquito breeding habitats to human populations varies depending on the specific geographic location and local conditions. In general, *Anopheles* mosquitoes tend to breed in areas near human settlements both in urban and rural settings and take advantage of readily available blood meals. The main vectors of malaria, which are *Anopheles gambiae* and *An. funestus* and *An. arabiesis*, transmit the causative parasites particularly *Plasmodium falciparum* and to a lesser extent, *P. vivax.* Specific mosquito species' presence and abundance varies within countries depending on local environmental factors. The transmission dynamics of *Anopheles* mosquito species are influenced by factors such as vector behavior, ecology, vector control interventions, host availability, and the prevalence of malaria parasites within the human population.

The contribution of domestic animals to *Anopheles* mosquito breeding and malaria transmission depends on local conditions, such as vector species, animal husbandry practices, and malaria prevalence in both humans and animals. Factors such as population movements, inadequate healthcare infrastructure, poverty, and limited access to effective prevention and treatment measures contribute to the persistence of malaria in the region. Efforts to interrupt malaria transmission in East Africa target both the mosquito vectors and the human hosts. Human behavior significantly impacts malaria transmission in the region. Outdoor activities during peak mosquito biting hours and inadequate use of preventive measures, such as insecticide-treated bed nets, increase the risk of mosquito bites and subsequently lead to malaria infection.

The climate, especially rainfall patterns and temperature affects both the mosquito and the malaria parasite's life cycle. Rainfall patterns affect the availability of breeding sites for mosquitoes when stagnant water from rainfall provides ideal conditions for mosquito larvae to thrive. The daily temperature variation influence their survival, development, and reproduction rates with higher temperatures leading to faster development rates of mosquitoes from egg to adult, resulting in more rapid mosquito population growth. Daily temperature variations also influence human behavior pertaining to use of bed nets where people may be less likely to sleep under bed nets during hot nights, leading to increased exposure to mosquito bites.

The sub-region faces several challenges in its efforts to control malaria. These challenges include the emergence of drug-resistant malaria parasites, insecticide-resistant mosquitoes, inadequate healthcare infrastructure, and limited resources for implementing comprehensive control programs. The lack of awareness about malaria prevention and treatment measures may also lead to delays in seeking appropriate healthcare, further exacerbating the disease's transmission. Overcoming these intervention challenges requires collaboration among researchers, policymakers, and local communities to develop context-specific and sustainable approaches for malaria control in East Africa. Additionally, continuous monitoring and adaptation of strategies are essential to address evolving challenges and ensure progress toward malaria elimination goals.

Acknowledgements

I acknowledge the support by my employer, Jaramogi Oginga Odinga University of Science and Technology (JOOUST), especially financially and granting me a portion of time within which I was able to contribute this chapter. I also wish to acknowledge the authors led by Victor A. Alegana for utilizing their map of *Plasmodium falciparum* prevalence in East Africa. I thank Wendy P.L.A. Davis for the thorough editorial work she rendered to this chapter.

Author details

Fred Anangwe Amimo
Jaramogi Oginga Odinga University of Science and Technology, Bondo, Kenya

*Address all correspondence to: amimofa@gmail.com

IntechOpen

© 2023 The Author(s). Licensee IntechOpen. This chapter is distributed under the terms of the Creative Commons Attribution License (http://creativecommons.org/licenses/by/3.0), which permits unrestricted use, distribution, and reproduction in any medium, provided the original work is properly cited.

References

[1] WHO. World Malaria Report 2018. Geneva: World Health Organization; 2018

[2] WHO. World Malaria Report 2020. World Health Organization. 2018. Available from: https://www.who.int/publications/i/item/9789240015791 [Accessed: September 15, 2021]

[3] Fontenille D, Simard F. Unraveling complexities in human malaria transmission dynamics in Africa through a comprehensive knowledge synthesis. Annual Review of Entomology. 2020;**65**:387-408

[4] Sachs JD, Melaney P. The economic and social burden of malaria. Nature. 2002;**415**:680-685

[5] WHO. Malaria Guidelines. Geneva: World Health Organization; 2023

[6] Deribew A, Alemseged F, Birhanu Z, Sena L, Tegegn A, Zeynudin A, et al. The effect of household heads training about environmental factors on long-lasting insecticidal net use in Ethiopia. BMC Public Health. 2012;**12**:914. DOI: 10.1186/1471-2458-12-914

[7] Mwangangi JM, Mbogo CM, Orindi BO, Muturi EJ, Midega JT, Nzovu J, et al. Shifts in malaria vector species composition and transmission dynamics along the Kenyan coast over the past 20 years. Malaria Journal. 2013;**12**:13. DOI: 10.1186/1475-2875-12-13

[8] Afrane YA, Zhou G, Lawson BW, Githeko AK, Yan G. Life-table analysis of *Anopheles arabiensis* in western Kenya highlands: Effects of land covers on larval and adult survivorship. The American Journal of Tropical Medicine and Hygiene. 2007;**77**(1):660-666. DOI: 10.4269/ajtmh.2007.77.660

[9] Coetzee M. Distribution of the African malaria vectors of the *Anopheles gambiae* complex. The American Journal of Tropical Medicine and Hygiene. 2004;**70**:105-109

[10] Cohen JM, Smith DL, Cotter C, Ward A, Yamey G, Sabot OJ, et al. Malaria resurgence: A systematic review and assessment of its causes. Malaria Journal. 2012;**11**:122. DOI: 10.1186/1475-2875-11-122

[11] Kweka EJ, Zhou G, Lee MC, Gilbreath TM 3rd, Mosha F, Munga S, et al. Evaluation of two methods of estimating larval habitat productivity in western Kenya highlands. Parasites & Vectors. 2011;**4**:110. DOI: 10.1186/1756-3305-4-110

[12] Kigozi R, Baxi SM, Gasasira A, Sserwanga A, Kakeeto S, Nasr S, et al. Indoor residual spraying of insecticide and malaria morbidity in a high transmission intensity area of Uganda. PLoS One. 2012;**7**(8):e42857. DOI: 10.1371/journal.pone.0042857

[13] Minakawa N, Sonye G, Mogi M, Githeko AK, Yan G. The effects of climatic factors on the distribution and abundance of malaria vectors in Kenya. Journal of Medical Entomology. 2002;**39**(3):833-841. DOI: 10.1603/0022-2585-39.6.833

[14] WHO/UNICEF. The Malaria Report 2005: Roll Back Malaria Monitoring and Evaluation. Geneva, Switzerland: UNICEF; 2005

[15] Beeson JG, Drew DR, Boyle MJ, Feng G, Fowkes FJI, Richards JS. Merozoite surface proteins in red blood cell invasion, immunity, and vaccines against malaria. FEMS Microbiology Reviews. 2016;**40**(3):343-372

[16] Zhou G, Minakawa N, Githeko AK, Yan G. Association between climate variability and malaria epidemics in the East African highlands. Proceedings of the National Academy of Sciences of the United States of America. 2004;**101**(51):2375-2380. DOI: 10.1073/pnas.0308714100

[17] Tusting LS, Rek JC, Arinaitwe E, Staedke SG, Kamya MR, Cano J, et al. Measuring socioeconomic inequalities in relation to malaria risk: A comparison of metrics in rural Uganda. The American Journal of Tropical Medicine and Hygiene. 2016;**94**(3):650-658. DOI: 10.4269/ajtmh.15-0547

[18] Walker M, Winskill P, Basanez MG, Mwangangi JM, Mbogo C, Beier JC, et al. Temporal and micro-spatial heterogeneity in the distribution of Anopheles vectors of malaria along the Kenyan coast. Parasites & Vectors. 2013;**6**:311. DOI: 10.1186/1756-3305-6-311

[19] Gething PW, Patil AP, Smith DL, Guerra CA, Elyazar IR, Johnston GL, et al. Hay SI: A new world malaria map: *Plasmodium falciparum* endemicity in 2010. Malaria Journal. 2011;**10**:378. DOI: 10.1186/1475-2875-10-378

[20] Okiro EA, Al-Taiar A, Reyburn H, Idro R, Berkley JA, Snow RW. Age patterns of severe paediatric malaria and their relationship to *Plasmodium falciparum* transmission intensity. Malaria Journal. 2009;**8**:4. DOI: 10.1186/1475-2875-8-4

[21] Githeko AK, Service MW, Mbogo CM, Atieli FK, Juma FO. Origin of blood meals in indoor and outdoor resting malaria vectors in western Kenya. Acta Tropica. 1994;**58**(3-4):307-316. DOI: 10.1016/0001-706x(94)90081-7

[22] Beier JC, Perkins PV, Onyango FK, Gargan TP, Oster CN, Whitmire RE, et al. Characterization of malaria transmission by *Anopheles* (Diptera: Culicidae) mosquitoes in western Kenya in preparation for malaria vaccine trials. Journal of Medical Entomology. 1990;**27**(6):570-577. DOI: 10.1093/jmedent/27.6.570

[23] Alegana VA, Macharia PM, Muchiri S, Mumo E, Oyugi E, Kamau A, et al. Plasmodium falciparum parasite prevalence in East Africa: Updating data for malaria stratification. PLOS Global Public Health. 7 Dec 2021;**1**(12):e0000014. DOI: 10.1371/journal.pgph.0000014

[24] Alegana VA, Macharia PM, Muchiri S, Mumo E, Oyugi E, Kamau A, et al. *Plasmodium falciparum* Parasite Prevalence in East Africa: Updating Data for Malaria Stratification2021. DOI: 10.1371/journal.pgph.0000014

[25] Kristan M, Abeku TA, Beard J, Okia M, Rapuoda B, Sang J, et al. Variations in entomological indices in relation to weather patterns and malaria incidence in East African highlands: Implications for epidemic prevention and control. Malaria Journal. 2008;**7**:231

[26] Smith T, Schellenberg JA, Hayes R. Attributable fraction estimates and case definitions for malaria in endemic areas. Statistics in Medicine. 1994;**13**(18):2345-2358. DOI: 10.1002/sim.4780131803

[27] Bousema T, Drakeley C. Epidemiology and infectivity of *Plasmodium falciparum* and *Plasmodium vivax* gametocytes in relation to malaria control and elimination. Clinical Microbiology Reviews. 2011;**24**(2):377-410. DOI: 10.1128/CMR.00051-10

[28] Kweka EJ, Zhou G, Munga S, Lee MC, Atieli HE, Nyindo M, et al. Anopheline mosquito species in Kenya: Ecological distribution and malaria

infection prevalence. Parasites & Vectors. 2015;**8**:328. DOI: 10.1186/s13071-015-0937-y

[29] Charlwood JD, Vij R, Billingsley PF. Dry season refugia of malaria-transmitting mosquitoes in a dry savannah zone of East Africa. The American Journal of Tropical Medicine and Hygiene. 2000;**62**:726-732

[30] Koenraadt CJ, Githeko AK, Takken W. The effects of rainfall and evapotranspiration on the temporal dynamics of *Anopheles gambiae* s.s. and Anopheles arabiensis in a Kenyan village. Acta Tropica. 2004;**90**:141-153. DOI: 10.1016/j.actatropica.2003.11.007

[31] Zhou G, Munga S, Minakawa N, Githeko AK, Yan G. Spatial relationship between adult malaria vector abundance and environmental factors in western Kenya highlands. The American Journal of Tropical Medicine and Hygiene. 2007;77:29-35

[32] WHO Malaria Report 2020. 20 Years of Global Progress & Challenges. 30 Nov 2020. ISBN 978-92-4-001579-1. Available from: https://www.who.int/publications/i/item/9789240015791

[33] Where Malaria Occurs. Global Health, Division of Parasitic Diseases and Malaria. 9 Apr 2020. Available from: https://www.cdc.gov/malaria/index.html

[34] Predicting the Effect of Seasonality on Malaria Transmission. Malaria Atlas Project. 2023. Available from: https://www.malariaatlas.org

[35] Hay SI, Guerra CA, Tatem AJ, Atkinson PM, Snow RW. Urbanization, malaria transmission and disease burden in Africa. Nature Reviews Microbiology. 2005;**3**(1):81-90. DOI: 10.1038/nrmicro1069

[36] Tiono AB, Ouedraogo A, Diarra A, Coulibaly SN, Soulama I, Konate AT, et al. Patterns of malaria morbidity and mortality in Dielmo, a periurban area of Senegal. Malaria Journal. 2018;**17**(1):422. DOI: 10.1186/s12936-018-2594-2

[37] Gillies MT, De Meillon B. The Anophelinae of Africa South of the Sahara (Ethiopian Zoogeographical Region). Vol. 54. 2nd edn. Johannesburg: South African Institute for Medical Research; 1968

[38] Malaria Surveillance, Monitoring & Evaluation: A Reference Manual. ISBN 978-92-4-156557-8 © World Health Organization. 2018

[39] President's Malaria Initiative (PMI) Impact Malaria. Washington, DC. 2018. Available from: www.pmi.gov/impact

[40] Mboera LE, Knols BG, Braks MA, Takken W. Comparison of carbon dioxide-baited trapping systems for sampling outdoor mosquito populations in Tanzania. Medical and Veterinary Entomology. 2000;**14**(3):257-263. DOI: 10.1046/j.1365-2915.2000.00242.x

[41] Ranson H, N'Guessan R, Lines J, Moiroux N, Nkuni Z, Corbel V. Pyrethroid resistance in African anopheline mosquitoes: What are the implications for malaria control? Trends in Parasitology. 2011;**27**(2):91-98. DOI: 10.1016/j.pt.2010.08.004

[42] Kiwuwa MS, Mufubenga P. Use of insecticide treated nets in a rural community in Wakiso district, Uganda. African Health Science. 2008;**8**(1):114-119

[43] Koenker HM, Yukich JO, Mkindi A, Mandike R, Brown N, Kilian A, et al. Value of a comprehensive malaria control intervention package: Approaches to measurement, short-term effects, and costs. American Journal of Tropical Medicine and Hygiene. 2013;**89**(1):88-99. DOI: 10.4269/ajtmh.12-0758

[44] Paaijmans KP, Blanford S, Bell AS, Blanford JI, Read AF, Thomas MB. Influence of climate on malaria transmission depends on daily temperature variation. Proceedings of the National Academy of Sciences. 2010;**107**(34):15135-15139. DOI: 10.1073/pnas.1006422107

[45] Lwetoijera DW, Kiware SS, Mageni ZD, Dongus S, Harris C, Devine GJ, et al. A need for better housing to further reduce indoor malaria transmission in areas with high bed net coverage. Parasites & Vectors. 2014;**7**(1):1-10. DOI: 10.1186/1756-3305-7-234

[46] Yukich JO, Chitnis N, Kenney L. Targeted coverage campaigns for universal bed net access in rural Tanzania: Analysis of spatially explicit data from an open cohort study. The Lancet Planetary Health. 2018;**2**(8):e367-e376. DOI: 10.1016/s2542-5196(18)30117-9

[47] WHO. Global Malaria Programme. Global technical strategy for malaria, 2016-2030. World Health Organization. 2015

Chapter 5

Complexity of Vector Control and Entomological Surveillance in Endemic Sentinel Sites of the National Malaria Control Program (NMCP) in the Democratic Republic of Congo (DRC)

Emery Metelo, Josue Zanga, Doudou Batumbo, Bien-aimé Mandja, Hyacinthe Lukoki, Arsène Bokulu, Trèsor Iluku, Narcisse Basosila, Emile Manzambi, Fiacre Agossa and Erick Mukomena

Abstract

In order to represent the different epidemiological facies that abound in the Democratic Republic of Congo (DRC), new sentinel sites were created. Before their operationalization, baseline evaluations of the bionomics and the insecticide resistance status of malaria vectors were conducted. Using Human Landing Catches (HLCs) and Pyrethrum Spray Catches (PSCs), sampled *Anopheles gambiae s.l.* were screened for the presence of *Plasmodium falciparum*. Larval surveys were organized to assess the sensitivity of wild *An. gambiae* to selected insecticides. Surveys on the community use of Insecticide-Treated Nets (ITNs), Surveys on the community use of Insecticide-Treated Nets (ITNs), were conducted. A total of 2238 *Anopheles* were collected. Including, 1802 (80.5%) by HLC and 436 (19.5%) by PSC. The majority of the samples were *An. gambiae* (98%) with very high average transmission entomological indices (density, Human Biting Rates (HBRs) and Entomological Inoculation Rates (EIRs)). These *An. gambiae* were resistant to selected insecticides at all sites. Households close to breeding sites were at high risk. Overall, ITN coverage was low (41.7%). Of these three sites, only Mweka presented a good coverage of 90%. Only Mweka presented a good coverage of 90%. The sentinel sites are located in the same epidemiological facies where the conditions for transmission of the disease and the incidence are identical. This transmission is ensured by *An. gambiae* with high resistance statuses vis-à-vis pyrethroids. The ecological choice is necessary for a good representation.

Keywords: *An. gambiae s.l.*, resistance, entomological indices, sentinel sites, DRC

1. Introduction

Malaria is a parasitosis that constitutes a global public health problem and is still endemic in many parts of the world with an estimated 247 million cases in 2021 [1]. It is particularly rife in Sub-Saharan Africa where 95% (234 million) of the global malaria cases and subsequently 96% (593,000) of all deaths occur. In this region of Africa, four countries (Nigeria 27%, the Democratic Republic of Congo (DRC) 12%, Uganda 5% and Mozambique 4%) pay a particularly heavy toll from malaria [1]. Nigeria and the DRC alone carry 39% of the global burden of malaria [1].

In the DRC, malaria remains a major public health problem, despite significant progress made [2, 3]. In 2021, the number of deaths associated with malaria was estimated at 22,729, of which 15,297 occurred of children under the age of 5, i.e., 67% [4, 5]. Around 97% of the population lives in areas with stable, endemic malaria transmission characterized by the equatorial and tropical facies [4]. This country has five distinct climatic zones (Equatorial zone, South tropical wet zone, South tropical dry zone, North tropical wet zone and Temperate tropical zone) [6]. The equatorial climate occupies the central basin and the tropical climate extends from north to south, thus occupying most of the country. The DRC stretches over an area of about 2,345,000 km^2, and it alone presents almost all the ecologies and bioclimatic strata encountered in Africa, from the Sahelian savannah regions to the equatorial forest regions [4]. This environmental heterogeneity makes combating malaria in the DRC particularly complex [6, 7]. Moreover, despite several rounds of mass distribution of ITNs, the country is struggling to achieve 60% ITN coverage [7].

This DRC has adhered to the World Health Organization's (WHO's) global technical strategy for the fight against malaria (2016–2030), which provides comprehensive technical guidance with the aim of reducing the incidence and mortality rates linked to malaria by at least 90% compared to 2015 reference year [1].

Large-scale use of ITNs offers good protection to populations at risk of malaria and has been the primary tool for vector control for nearly 40 years [8]. Taking this global strategy into account, for almost a decade the DRC has opted for building universal coverage of malaria control interventions within the National Strategic Plan (NSP) [4]. The current NSP adopted at the national level is aligned with the global technical strategy for the fight against malaria, with the objectives of reducing the rate of morbidity and mortality linked to malaria by at least 40% by the end of 2023 with coverage ≥80% in ITNs [4].

One of the guiding principles the NSP has set itself is the implementation of vector control based on evidence and convincing results [4]. To do this, the National Malaria Control Program (NMCP) relies on data from routine systematic surveys and studies [4, 7, 9] requiring the establishment of sentinel sites. Together, these sentinel sites generate inexpensive, complete and quality data [4]. They are distributed according to the health subdivision, Health Division (HD), Health Zone (HZ) and Health Area (HA), which is similar to the administrative subdivision (province, territory, community, village) seen elsewhere.

Parasitological, pharmacological and environmental data are needed to assess the evolution of malaria [4] and this guided how sentinel surveillance sites were created and located across the country on the basis of the Health Division (HD). Sentinel sites correspond to health surveillance zones where parasitological and entomological surveys are carried out to provide basic data for evaluating malaria control activities, and which represent the Province Health Division (PHD).

Before decentralization in 2010, the DRC had 11 provinces giving 11 sentinel sites. After decentralization, 26 provinces were obtained. Thus, the DRC will gradually add 15 new sites corresponding to one site in each of the 26 Provincial Health Divisions (PHDs) [10]. These sentinel sites represent the different epidemiological facies of malaria transmission found in the DRC.

It is important to note that the distribution of each *Anopheles* species relies on ecological characteristics favorable to their reproduction and multiplication [11, 12]. In the DRC, the most encountered vectors are *Anopheles gambiae*, *Anopheles funestus*, *Anopheles nili*, *Anopheles moucheti* and *Anopheles paludis* [4]. These species are not evenly distributed in all PHDs.

Surveys examining vector bionomics (behaviors including host preference, host-seeking, peak activity period as well as larval site characteristics) and insecticide resistance (IR) monitoring are carried out in the various sentinel sites for evidence that helps the NMCP choose the most appropriate vector control tools. The emergence of IR in the African region raises many questions about the ongoing effectiveness of ITNs in helping to reduce the incidence of malaria [8]. Increasing evidence of *Anopheles* resistance to different classes of insecticides is reported by several authors [9, 13, 14]. Thus, it is necessary that the choice of sentinel sites take into account the ecology and the bionomics of the vectors, as well as the profiles of the *Anopheles* vis-à-vis the insecticides used.

The current choice of NMCP sentinel sites is based on administrative criteria alone and does not address the biodiversity of vector species and various epidemic facies. Indeed, the work of Rahm and Vermilin [15] on the distribution of anopheline species in all Congolese territories identified 66 species of *Anopheles*, whereas Watsenga et al.'s [9] work, based on sentinel sites in the DRC, identified fewer species. Yet, there is evidence elsewhere (Cameroon) that a greater diversity of species can be identified when the choice of sentinel sites is based on ecological criteria [16].

To enable the new sentinel sites to fully play their role by providing reliable data and reflecting the local reality of malaria transmission, this pilot study was carried out to assess entomological surveillance in the nine additional sentinel sites. Only four sites, namely Boende in the Province of Tshuapa, Lisala in the Province of Mongala, Mweka in Kasai and Nyakunde in Ituri, were selected.

The present study aims to contribute to our understanding of the local epidemiology of malaria by identifying vector species, determining entomological parameters (species, density, HBR and EIR) and the profile of *An. gambiae s.l.'s* susceptibility to the usual insecticides and the factors modulating the transmission of malaria in the sentinel sites.

2. Complexity of vector control and entomological surveillance in endemic sentinel sites of the NMCP in DRC

2.1 Methods

2.1.1 Study sites

The study was conducted in four new sentinel sites, from June 17 to July 17, 2019 for the first three sites (Boende, Lisala and Nyakunde) and from October 15 to November 15, 2019 for the Mweka site (**Figure 1**) by three teams of entomologists from Laboratory of Bio-ecology and Vector Control at the Kinshasa School of Public

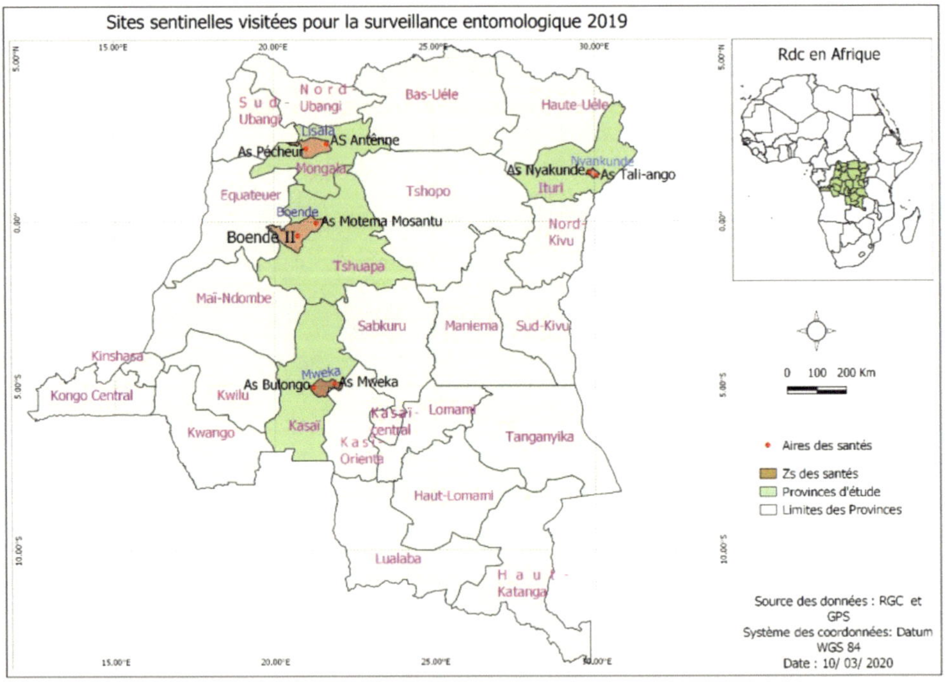

Figure 1.
Sentinel mosquito collection sites (in green, the provinces and in red the capture point).

Sentinel site	Province	[1]GPS coordinates	Selected [2]HA	Frequency and period of data collection	Climatic zone
Bende	Tshuapa	0°16′47″S	Motema mosantu	4 times during a week (June or July 2019)	Equatorial
		20°52′39″E	Kimbangu II	4 times during a week (June or July 2019)	
Lisala	Mongala	2°9′0″ N	Antenne	4 times during a week (June or July 2019)	Equatorial
		21°31′0″ E	Fisherman	4 times during a week (June or July 2019)	
Nyakunde	Ituri	1°25′60″ N	Nyakunde	4 times during a week (June or July 2019)	Equatorial
		30°1′60″ E	Birinyama	4 times during a week (June or July 2019)	
Mweka	Kasaï	4°50′60″S	Mweka 1	4 times during a week (October or November 2019)	[3]S Too w
		2°34′0″ E	Bulongo	4 times during a week (October or November 2019)	

[1]*GPS, Global Positioning System.*
[2]*HA, Health Area.*
[3]*S Too w, South Tropical Wet.*

Table 1.
Entomological sentinel site location, period of data collection and climatic zone.

Health (BIOLAV-KSPH). Location of entomological sentinel sites and frequency of sensitivity testing and trapping to determine human bite rates are given in **Table 1**.

2.1.1.1 Boende

Boende is located in the Province of Tshuapa, on the Tshuapa and Lomami rivers, east of Mbandaka, 1400 km north-east of the capital Kinshasa. It is served by Route Nationale 8.

2.1.1.2 Lisala

Lisala is located in Mongala province, on the right bank of the Congo River, in a forested area with an equatorial climate. It lies 2650 km north-east of Kinshasa and is served by the Route Nationale 6.

2.1.1.3 Nyakunde

Nyakunde is the seat of the Andisoma chiefdom of the Bira, located some 30 km south-west of Bunia, in the Irumu territory, Ituri district, Orientale Province in northeastern Democratic Republic of Congo. It comprises three regions with distinct climatic characteristics: a very rainy region like the equatorial basin, an intermediate zone where rainfall decreases during the dry season like the tropical zone, and a territory with little rainfall but alternating between the two seasons.

2.1.1.4 Mweka

Mweka is a decentralized entity in the Province of Kasai in the Democratic Republic of Congo. Located in a savannah zone with a humid tropical climate with two seasons (dry from May to September and rainy September to December), the territory is characterized by a slightly warm temperature with a maximum estimated at 27°C. The climatic elements (temperature and rainfall) for all three sites sampled at different stations (Lisala, Tshuapa and Tshikapa) are shown in **Figure 2**.

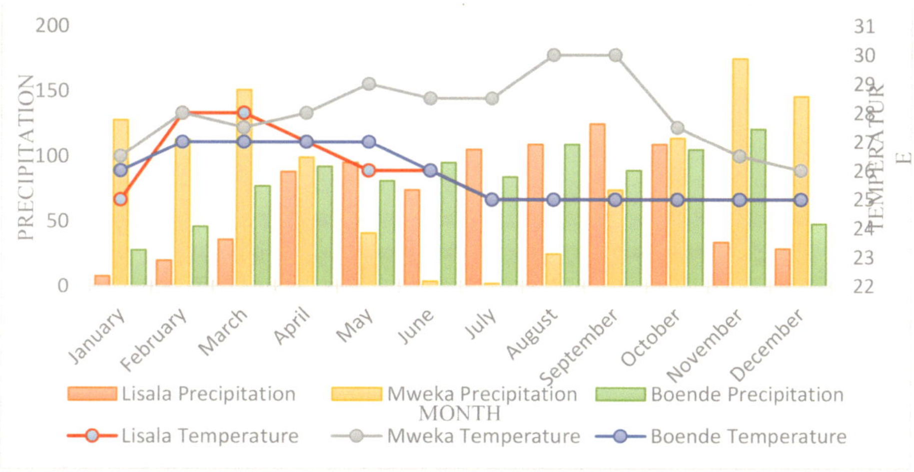

Figure 2.
Ombrothermic curve of Mweka, Lisala and Boende in 2019 (source: Lisala, Tshuapa and Tshikapa weather station).

2.1.2 Study population and sampling technique

The statistical unit of the study was the *Anopheles* mosquito specimens, which were collected from selected houses using a four-stage probability sampling technique:

- Four sentinel sites corresponding to four Provincial Health Divisions (PHDs) were randomly selected from nine newly created NMCP sentinel sites.

- Two health areas (HAs) were randomly selected from those carrying out sentinel surveillance in the site.

- Two villages were selected among all those constituting the selected health area.

- Ten houses per village were selected, according to the World Health Organization (WHO) recommendation, to have a good representation [17].

However, one of the surveys was underway and it was possible to sample only in three sites (Boende, Lisala and Mweka) out of the four initially planned, i.e., a total of 60 houses instead of the 80. Unfortunately, security threats at the sentinel sites within Nyakunde prevented the surveys from going ahead as intended. Thus, this site was removed from our analyses.

2.1.3 Data collection study procedure

2.1.3.1 Mosquito collection

2.1.3.1.1 Larva collection

Larvae and pupae of *An. gambiae s.l.* were collected from different larval sites. After sorting, the selected larvae were reared in tanks covered with mosquito nets and then kept under conditions likely to favor the emergence of mosquitoes, without contamination of the rearing by external mosquitoes and without infestation of the environment. The daily monitoring of the farm consisted in counting the numbers of larvae in each tank, on the one hand, and living and dead imagoes in each cage, on the other hand [18].

2.1.3.1.2 Adult mosquitoes (anopheles)

Two collection methods were used: Capture by indoor spraying with pyrethrums (PSCs) allowing the residual density of resting anophelines and their trophic states to be established; and human landing catches (HLCs) to assess the risk of infective/human/night bites, *Anopheles* behavior and the cycle of aggression (peak biting).

2.1.3.1.3 Human landing catches (HLCs)

Human landing catches (HLCs) were conducted in 10 houses per village from 6 p.m. to 6 a.m., and the data reported cover only 12 h of nocturnal captures. Thus, in each village, 10 houses were selected for capture, giving a total of 20 houses per site and 60 houses for all sites. As mentioned above, the Nyakunde data were not taken into account. Four mosquito collectors were assigned to each house, i.e., two outdoor and two indoor. After sorting the mosquitoes morphologically to identify the anophelines in the field, the mosquitoes were individually preserved in Eppendorf tubes with silica gel and brought back to the BIOLAV/KSPH laboratory for further analysis (identification, determination of infectivity and WHO Tube Pass sensitivity test) [19].

2.1.3.1.4 Capture by indoor pyrethrum spray (PSC)

The PSC was carried out by spraying a pyrethrum-based insecticide in 10 non-HLC houses between 6 and 10 a.m. after removing cooking utensils, drinks and food. White sheets were spread out on the floor in all rooms of the house and spraying began outside the house, in front of doors and windows, then inside. A commercially available pyrethroid spray (Baygon, Bayer) was sprayed in the house and doors were closed for 15 min. After which, doors and windows were opened to collect mosquitoes that had fallen onto the sheets. Female mosquitoes were classified according to four trophic statuses (unfed, freshly fed, half-gravid and gravid) [17, 20].

2.1.4 Household survey

The household surveys were carried out in each of the houses where the mosquitoes were captured. Household heads were interviewed based on the questions administered in the Malaria Indicator Surveys (MIS). The questionnaire included questions on sociodemographic status, the notion of fever in children under 5 years of age, the use or not of mosquito nets and the physical condition of ITNs. The type of construction materials of the houses (blackberries and roofs) was also characterized in order to determine the quality of the habitat allowing the access or not of the mosquitoes [7].

2.1.5 Data and studies procedure

2.1.5.1 Morphological identification of Culicidae

The mosquitoes were sorted based on morphological criteria to gender and sex in the field. They were then stored individually in Eppendorf tubes with silica gel and sent to the entomology laboratory of the Kinshasa School of Public Health (KSPH). Once in the laboratory, morphological identification under the microscope was conducted using dichotomous keys [21, 22].

2.1.5.2 Insecticide susceptibility tests and synergist bioassays

Sensitivity tests were carried out on wild populations of *Anopheles* in each of the four sentinel sites selected. They made it possible to better know the levels of sensitivity of the vectors to the two Pyrethroids (Alphacypermethrin and Deltamethrin). And in the event of resistance to pyrethroids, a pre-exposure to Piperonyl Butoxide (PBO) was carried out for the search for oxidases. The effectiveness of these compounds was compared with that of DDT and Bendiocarb, to detect the existence or not of cross-resistance between the three chemical families. And this insecticide's effectiveness was measured according to their knockdown effect (Kdt_{50} and Kdt_{95}) and the mortality they cause after 24 h of observation.

Larval collections were made in each study site using larval dippers. Larval sampling was done in transient, sun-exposed puddles to maximize the likelihood of sampling *An. gambiae s.l.*. Larvae were subsequently transported to a field insectary for rearing. Emerging adult mosquitoes were provided with sugar solution until they were used for insecticide susceptibility tests [9].

Adult females 2–5 days old were selected and tested according to the WHO protocol [18]. The tests were carried out with the papers impregnated with insecticides from the WHO Kit composed of four types of insecticides and the PBO synergist of different concentrations: Deltamethrin 0.05%, Alphacypermethrin 0.05%, Bendiocarb 0.1%, DDT 4% and PBO 5%. And the effectiveness of insecticide was measured according to their knockdown effect for 60 min of contact and the mortality they cause after 24 h of observation.

The tests were carried out in accordance with the general conditions of the test procedures recommended by the WHO, particularly with regard to: temperature (between 23 and 27°C), relative humidity (between 70 and 90%), the age of the adult female mosquitoes (2 to 5 days), the number of times an insecticide-treated paper should be used (Not more than 6 times/At most 150 mosquitoes per paper for pyrethroids), the qualities and the number of uses of control test papers [18].

For each insecticide retained, four test replications, each involving 25 mosquitoes, were carried out. The first series of tests was carried out to observe the behavior of *An. gambiae s.l.* after 60 min of contact with insecticides. The numbers of mosquitoes shocked after 10, 15, 20, 30, 40, 50 and 60 min of exposure or contact with the insecticide were recorded, in order to calculate the shock effect (Kdt_{50} and Kdt_{95}). Twenty-five mosquitoes were used for the negative control. After exposure, mosquitoes were transferred to clean holding tubes and provided with sugar solution. Mortality was recorded 24 h after exposure.

In the event of resistance to pyrethroids, a second series of tests was carried out with anophelines pre-exposed to PBO for 60 min.

The test results were interpreted according to the WHO criteria [18]:

- Susceptible (S), if mortality is between 98 and 100%;
- Probably Resistant (PR), if mortality is between 90 and 97%.
- Resistant (R), if mortality is less than 90%;

2.1.5.3 Determination of the infectivity rate by the enzyme-linked immunosorbent assay (ELISA)-plasmodium falciparum circumsporozoite protein (ELISA-CSP) pf technique

After morphological identification, a subsample of individually stored *An. gambiae s.l.* collected by HLC were analyzed at the Institut National de la Recherche Biomédicale (INRB). The *An. gambiae s.l.* female were ground for analysis in the pf CSP ELISA test according to the Wurtz protocol.

The sporozoite index (SI) was determined after ELISA-CSP to detect the presence of the circumsporozoite protein of *P. falciparum*. However, after grinding Blocking Buffer (BB-IGEPAL®) using a pestle, the Pf monoclonal antibodies (mAb Pf) were fixed on the microplates, and the ground material was brought into contact with the mAb Pf. In addition, the enzyme-coupled conjugate (mAb capture, peroxidase) was added before adding the enzyme substrate (hydrogen peroxide (H_2O_2)). Then, the reading was made with an ELISA reader at 405 nm.

2.1.5.4 Determination of entomological indices of transmission

2.1.5.4.1 Indoor resting density (IRD)

Density of resting mosquitoes inside houses was estimated by the total number of female mosquitoes resting indoors on the total number of houses inspected.

2.1.5.4.2 Human biting rate (HBR)

This rate designates the number of mosquito bites received by a person during one night (bite/human/night). It was estimated on the basis of the number of *Anopheles* caught on human bait, from 6 p.m. to 6 a.m.

2.1.5.4.3 Entomological inoculation rate (EIR)

The entomological inoculation rate (EIR) represents the average number of infective bites per human per night (ib/h/n). It is calculated as follows:

$$EIR = HBR \times \text{Sporozoite index}\,(\%) / 100. \qquad (1)$$

2.1.6 Data analysis

Data were entered using Microsoft Excel® 2016. Statistical analyses of study data were performed using R® software in version 4.1.2. A statistical analysis was carried out on certain parameters with the usual statistical tests.

The data were essentially summarized in the form of a proportion because it was mainly necessary to calculate the entomological indices. Additionally, data were summarized in tables and graphs using Microsoft Excel® 2016 and R® 4.1.2. As the Shapiro test and the quantile-quantile (QQ) graph showed that the distribution of our data was not normal, it was more the nonparametric tests that were used in the rest of the analyses. The results obtained in the six health areas during the different surveys were compared using Kruskal-Wallis tests on the one hand, for the comparison of the medians and Fisher exact to compare the proportions. To determine factors associated with anopheline density, a nonparametric Theil-Sen regression model was used. Before performing the regression, exploratory univariate analyses were performed to identify independent variables significantly associated with anopheline density. A two-sided alpha level of 0.05 was considered statistically significant.

2.2 Results

2.2.1 Mosquito species composition and abundance

A total of 6697 mosquitoes were collected by HLC and PSC. *Culex* were most abundant with 4459 (66.58%), compared to 2238 *Anopheles* (33.41%). Of the 2238 *Anopheles* collected, 1802 were collected by HLC and 436 by PSC.

Of the 436 *Anopheles* collected, *An. gambiae s.l.* was predominant with 430 specimens (98%). *An. funestus* and *Anopheles ziemani* were poorly represented with, respectively, five and one specimens (1.15 and 0.23%) (**Figure 3**). Mweka presented a higher abundance of 156 *Anopheles* specimens (35.78%) than the other two sites.

In view of the observations made by HLC, it emerges from **Figure 4** that 1802 mosquitoes were captured in the three sites. Indeed, *An. gambiae s.l.* showed a

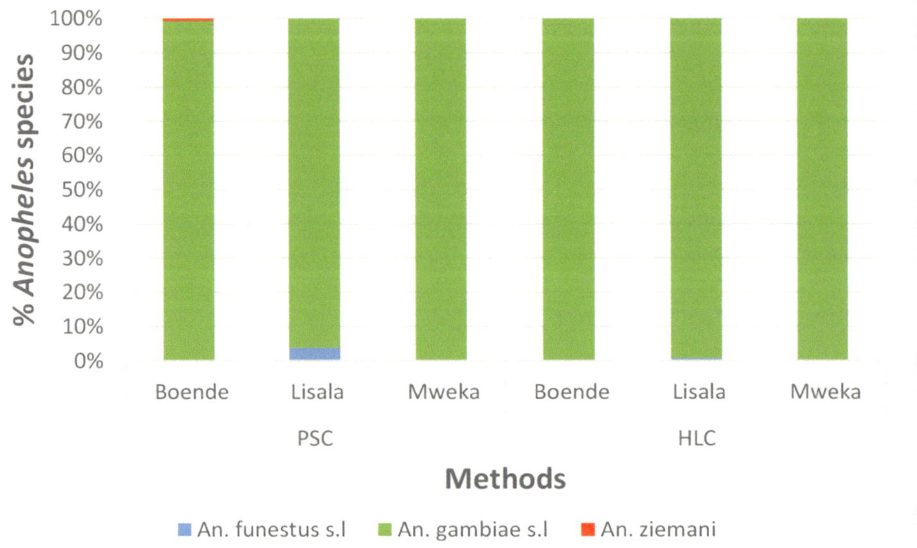

Figure 3.
Distribution of anopheles collected by PSC and HLC according to three sentinel sites.

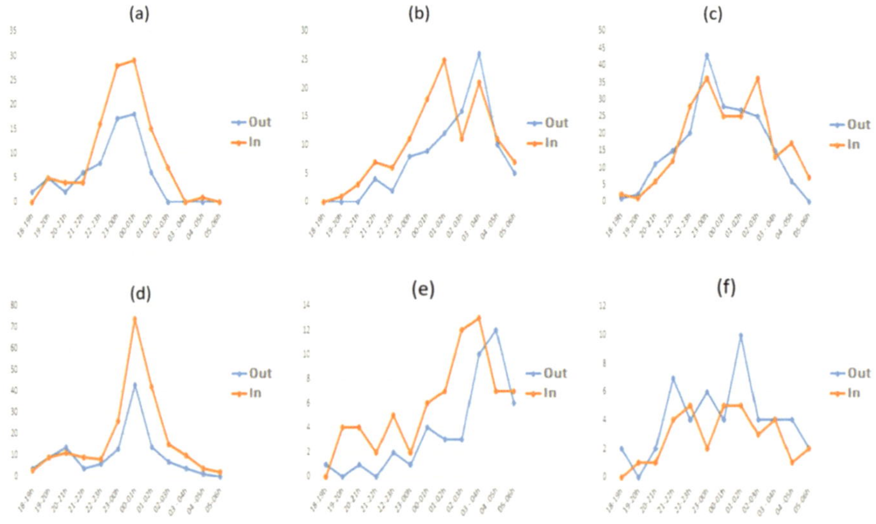

Figure 4.
Biting time of an. Gambiae s.l. collected by HLC according to sentinel sites. (a) Lisala (As pêcheur), (b) Boende (As motema-mosantu), (c) Mweka (As Mweka), (d) Lisala (As antenne), (e) Boende (As Boende II), (f) Mweka (As Mweka). Out = outdoor; In = indoor.

remarkable abundance of 1796 specimens (or 99.67%). The remaining two species (*An. funestus* and *An. ziemani*) were poorly represented with five and one specimens (i.e., 0.28 and 0.06%) (**Figure 3**). The Mweka site was the most abundant site in*Anopheles*, with 664 specimens (36.85%).

2.2.2 Determination of entomological parameters

2.2.2.1 PSC collection

With regard to the results presented in **Table 2**, the Resting Density Index (RDI) and the Indirect Human Biting Rate (IHBR) observed vary greatly from one site to another, and even from one village to another. Thus, the average values observed varied from 4.9 to 10 *An.*/house for the RDI and from 0.08 to 1.55*An.* fed/human/night for the indirect bite.

The highest and lowest RDIs were, respectively, observed in the Buza district (Boende II/Kimbangu) and Hôpital (Motema-Mosantu) from the Boende site (Tshuapa) with 10 and 4.9*An.* female/house, respectively.

As for indirect Human Biting Rate, the Buza district (Boende II/Kimbangu) presented the highest indirect bite rate next to the 3C district (Antenne), which presented the lowest indirect bite rate with, respectively, 1.55 and 0.08*An.* fed/human/night.

2.2.2.2 Human landing catch (HLC)

2.2.2.2.1 Biting time

Overall, anopheline biting activity started very early at 6 p.m., initially increasing gradually until 10 p.m. where the numbers captured increased at a higher rate before peaking between 24 a.m. and 2 a.m. The exception was Bulongo village where biting activity peaked notably later at 2 a.m. (indoors) and numbers captured began to decrease around 5 a.m. (**Figure 4**). The behavior of *Anopheles* sp. was more endophagic at all sites.

2.2.3 Entomological clues of transmission

It appears from **Table 3** that the average of the entomological indices of transmission (density, HBR, SI and EIR) was high and varied from one site to another. High

Sentinel site, Capture district or village (Health area)		**RDI* (*An.*/house)**	**I HBR* (*An.* fed/human/night)**
Boende (Tshuapa)	Hôpital (Motema mosantu)	4.9	0.51
	Buza (Boende II/Kimbangu)	10	1.55
Lisala (Mongala)	Lokele (Pêcheur)	7.5	0.27
	3C (Antenne)	6.1	0.08
Mweka (Kasai)	Congo I (Mweka)	9	0.98
	Village Bulongo (Bulongo)	6.1	0.92

**RDI: Relative density indoor (mean numbers of Anopheles per house). IHBI: Indirect Human Biting Rate (Anopheles fed/human/night).*

Table 2.
Entomological evaluation indices by PSC in sentinel sites.

Sites	Health area	Density An./ House	*HBR outdoor b/h/n	HBR indoor b/h/n	HBR b/h/n	*SI%	*EIR ib./h/n
Tshuapa Boende	Motema mosantu	4.9	9.3	12.3	10.8	11.5	1.2
	Boende II	10	4.3	6.9	5.6		
Mongala Lisala	Pêcheur	7.5	6.4	10.9	8.7	9.8	0.85
	Antenne	6.1	11.9	21.3	16.6		
Kasai Mweka	Mweka 1	9	19.3	20.3	19.8	13.8	2.73
	Bulongo	6.1	4.3	6.9	5.6		
Mean		7.3	9.3	13.1	11.2	11.7	1.59

**HBR: Human Biting Rate (bite/human/night); SI: sporozoite index; EIR: entomological inoculation rate (infective bites/human/night).*

Table 3.
Synthesis of entomological indices of transmission.

density was recorded at Tshuapa Boende in Boende II health area (10 *Anopheles*/house), followed by Kasai Mweka in Mweka 1 health area (9 *Anopheles*/house), and low density was recorded in Tshuapa Boende in the Motema-Mosantu health area (4.9 years/house). The HBR was more recorded indoor (13.1 b/h/n) against 9.3 b/h/n outdoor. However, in Kasai Mweka in the health area of Mweka 1, the high rate of bites was recorded (19.8 b/h/n) and the same EIR (2.73 ib./h/n).

2.2.4 Anopheles susceptibility profile of gambiae s.l. against common insecticides

The results of WHO susceptibility tests carried out on wild populations of *An. gambiae s.l.* in the four sites (Tshuapa/Boende, Mongala/Lisala, Mweka/Kasaï and Ituri/Nyakunde) to the two pyrethroids (Alphacypermethrin and Deltamethrin), to the organochlorines (DDT) and to the carbamates (Bendiocarb) are recorded in **Figure 5**.

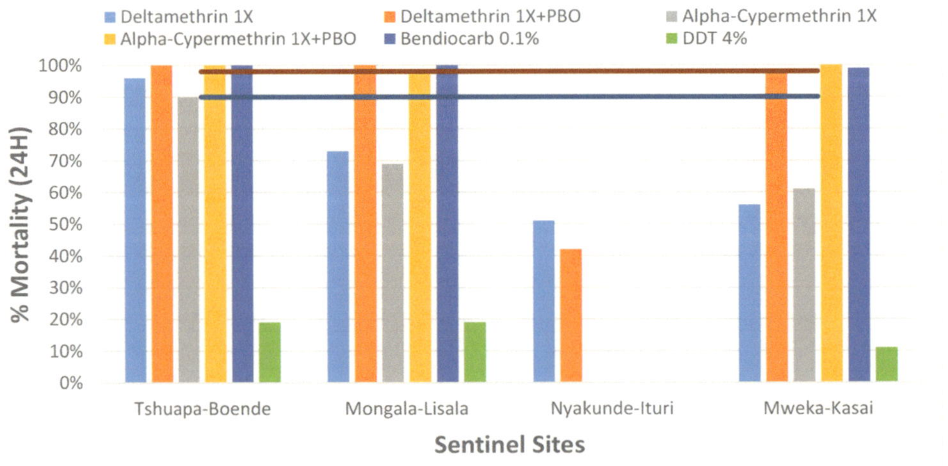

Figure 5.
Percentage mortality of an. Gambiae s.l. after pre-exposure to PBO followed by permethrin 1X and Alphacypermethrin 1X in WHO tube tests in four sites.

Susceptibility tests in indicated generally reveal that, across all collection sites, *An. gambiae s.l.* showed resistance (≤90%) of varying degrees to Alphacypermethrin and Deltamethrin. Separately, Deltamethrin mortality was slightly elevated at all sites in contrast to that of Alphacypermethrin. After pre-exposure of *An. gambiae s.l.* to PBO, the efficacy of Deltamethrin and Alphacypermethrin was fully restored at all sites to 98–100%.

Figure 5 shows that *An. gambiae s.l.* tested were more resistant to DDT with very low mortality of 11% in Mweka and 19% tied in Boende and Lisala. Only Bendiocarb was 100% effective at all sites.

Table 4 presents the analysis that determined the Kdt_{50} and Kdt_{95}, the value of these two parameters Kdt (knockdown time) corresponds to the time after which,

Sites	Insecticides	n	Kdt_{50} (min) IC 95%	Kdt_{95} (minute) IC 95%	Mortality 24 h (%)	Statut*
Tshuapa-Boende	Deltamethrine 0,05%	100	27,8 (26,2–29,4)	44,7 (41,9--48,3)	96	PR
	Deltamethrine 0,05% + PBO 5%	100	27,2 (26,0--28,5)	39,3 (37,3--42,1)	100	S
	Alphacypermethrine 0,5%	100	28,9 (26,5--31,2)	49.6(45.6--53.3)	90	R
	Alphacypermethrine 0,5% + PBO 5%	100	26,1 (25,2--27,0)	39,7 (38,1--41,8)	100	S
	DDT 4%	100	n/a	n / a	19	R
Mongala-Lisala	Deltamethrine 0,05%	100	37,3 (29,7–47,46)	n/a	73	R
	Deltamethrine 0,05% + PBO 5%	100	19.1 (16.7–21.1)	32,4 (28,1–40,3)	100	S
	Alphacypermethrine 0,5%	100	42,1 (35,5–51,3)	n/a	69	R
	Alphacypermethrine 0,5% + PBO 5%	100	20,8 (15,8--27,7)	37,1 (29,5--59,3)	98	S
	DDT 4%	100	n/a	n/a	19	R
Nyakunde-Ituri	Deltamethrine 0,05%	100	n/a	n/a	51	R
	Alphacypermethrine 0,5%	100	n/a	n/a	42	R
Mweka/Kasaï	Deltamethrine 0,05%	100	47,68 (44,5–51,6)	n/a	56	R
	Deltamethrine 0,05% + PBO 5%	100	23,5 (21,3–25,9)	43,6 (37,7–54,2)	98	S
	A	100	47,68 (44,5–51,6)	50,3 (45,9–56,1)	61	R
	Alphacypermethrine 0.,5% + PBO 5%	100	18,8 (16,9–20,6)	34,5 (29,9–42,6)	100	S
	DDT 4%	100	n/a	n/a	11	R

**R = resistance (24 h mortality ≤90%); S = sensibility (mortality 24 h 98–100%), RP = Resistance probability (mortality 24 h between 90 and 97%), n/a = not available.*

Table 4.
Knockdown time of an. Gambiae s.l. after 60 min exposure to insecticides and mortality after 24 h.

respectively, 50 and 95% of *An. gambiae s.l.* were knocked out after 60 min of insecticide contact. Kdt_{50} and Kdt_{95} have never been reached in all sites with DDT. The Kdt_{50} with Deltamethrin and Alphacypermethrin was not reached in the only site of Nyakunde and elsewhere, it was reached late.

Kdt_{95} with Deltamethrin and Alphacypermethrin was reached with difficulty and late at the Tshuapa/Boende site, respectively, at 44.7 min 95% confidence interval (CI) (41.9–48.3 min) and 49.6 min 95% CI (45.6–53.3 min). After pre-exposure to PBO, the efficacy of these two pyrethroids was restored and Kdt_{50} and Kdt_{95} were reached.

It is observed in Mweka, Kdt_{95} was not available to Deltamethrin and reached late forAlphacypermethrin by 50.3 (45.9–56.1) min, which reflected a high degree of resistance of *An. gambiae s.l.* to these two pyrethroids. However, in Nyakunde, Kdt_{95} was not available to Deltamethrin and Alphacypermethrin.

2.2.5 Infectivity rate

Sporozoite rates for all three sentinel sites are presented of 440 *An. gambiae s.l.* analyzed, the mean sporozoite rate in all sites being 11.6% (95% CI 3.4–5.2) for *An. gambiae s.l.* Moreover, sporozoite rates were relatively low at all sites. The lowest sporozoite rate was observed in Lisala at 9.8% (95% CI 1.1–4.6) and the highest at Mweka at 13.1 (95% CI 1.1–4.6).

2.2.6 Determination of factors modulating malaria transmission in sentinel sites

Table 5 shows that in the Antenne health area, out of the 10 houses surveyed, no engorged *Anopheles* were found, whereas the median value was higher in Motema-Mosantu, Boende 2 and Pêcheur. The difference in the medians in the six health areas is statistically significant ($p = 0.038$). The distance between houses and larval sites was shorter in the health area of Motema-Mosantu compared to the other health areas ($p < 0.001$). The quality of mosquito nets shows a significant difference between HAs ($p < 0.001$), with 0 and 1% for good quality of mosquito nets in Antenne and Mweka 1 HAs. The survey showed a difference in the proportions of metallic houses ($p < 0.001$), with 0% in AS Pêcheur, Bulongo, Mweka 1 and Boende 2 (**Table 5**). Possession of ITNs was very low in Lisala and Boende at 15 and 20%, respectively, and in Mweka there was good coverage of 90% with an average possession in the sites of 41.7%.

Table 6 shows that the anopheline density, according to our data, is significantly lower for houses located far from breeding larval sites (protective role because the odds ratio is less than 1). The other two variables were not statistically significant. The anopheline density with engorgement, according to our data, is significantly high for houses with a high number of ITNs.

The exponential of these coefficients gives the odds ratio, the distance between the household and the breeding site; the number of people in the household; and house type.

2.3 Discussion

2.3.1 Identification of vector species

After the staggered capture over the duration of the study, three species of *Anopheles* were identified overall but with a remarkably high density of *An. gambiae s.l.* found at all sites. However, according to Mouchet et al. [23], the different species of *Anopheles* exploit a wide variety of water collections as roosts, in particular the residual pools of

Variables	A	Pêcheur	Bulongo	Mweka_1	Boende_2	Motema_ Mosantu	Ooverall	Test
Anopheles_ density (Count)	10	10	10	10	10	10	60	Kruskal --Wallis (0.353)
Median (IQR)	2.50 (6.25)	3.50 (10.50)	2.00 (3.50)	1.50 (6.50)	4.00 (11.75)	6.50 (8.75)	3.00(8.00)	
Inphed (Count)	10	10	10	10	10	10	60	Kruskal --Wallis (0.038)
Median (IQR)	0.00 (0.00)	3.00 (5.75)	2.00 (0.75)	1.50 (4.00)	4.00 (6.75)	1.50 (2.75)	2.00(3.25)	
Household_ persons	10	10	10	10	10	10	60	Kruskal --Wallis (0.047)
Median (IQR)	3.50 (2.00)	4.50 (3.75)	5.50 (3.25)	7.00 (6.25)	5.00 (2.25)	8.00 (5.50)	5.00(4.00)	
Dist_house_ hablarva	10	10	10	10	10	10	60	Kruskal --Wallis (<0.001)
Median (IQR)	62.50 (71.50)	35.00 (27.50)	42.50 (17.50)	50.00 (27.50)	50.00 (17.50)	8.00 (1.00)	40.00 (36.25)	
ITN_Possession (%)	10 (16.67%)	10 (16.67%)	10 (16.67%)	10 (16.67%)	10 (16.67%)	10 (16.67%)	60	Fisher exact (0.152)
Yes	6 (40.00%) (60.00%)	2 (13.33%) (20.00%)	1 (6.67%) (10.00%)	2 (13.33%) (20.00%)	1 (6.67%) (10.00%)	3 (20.00%) (30.00%)	15 (100.00%) (25.00%)	
No	4 (8.89%) (40.00%)	8 (17.78%) (80.00%)	9 (20.00%) (90.00%)	8 (17.78%) (80.00%)	9 (20.00%) (90.00%)	7 (15.56%) (70.00%)	45 (100.00%) (75.00%)	
ITN_condition (%)	10 (16.67%)	10 (16.67%)	10 (16.67%)	10 (16.67%)	10 (16.67%)	10 (16.67%)	60	Fisher exact (<0.001)
Bad	10 (28.57%) (100.00%)	7 (20.00%) (70.00%)	1 (2.86%) (10.00%)	9 (25.71%) (90.00%)	1 (2.86%) (10.00%)	7 (20.00%) (70.00%)	35 (100.00%) (58.33%)	
Good	0 (0.00%) (0.00%)	3 (12.00%) (30.00%)	9 (36.00%) (90.00%)	1 (4.00%) (10.00%)	9 (36.00%) (90.00%)	3 (12.00%) (30.00%)	25 (100.00%) (41.67%)	
Fever (cCount (%))	10 (16.67%)	10 (16.67%)	10 (16.67%)	10 (16.67%)	10 (16.67%)	10 (16.67%)	60	Fisher exact (0.114)

Variables	A	Pêcheur	Bulongo	Mweka_1	Boende_2	Motema_ Mosantu	Ooverall	Test
Yes	8 (20.00%) (80.00%)	7 (17.50%) (70.00%)	7 (17.50%) (70.00%)	3 (7.50%) (30.00%)	6 (15.00%) (60.00%)	9 (22.50%) (90.00%)	40 (100.00%) (66.67%)	
No	2 (10.00%) (20.00%)	3 (15.00%) (30.00%)	3 (15.00%) (30.00%)	7 (35.00%) (70.00%)	4 (20.00%) (40.00%)	1 (5.00%) (10.00%)	20 (100.00%) (33.33%)	
House_type (%)	10 (16.67%)	10 (16.67%)	10 (16.67%)	10 (16.67%)	10 (16.67%)	10 (16.67%)	60	Fisher exact (<0.001)
s	0 (0.00%) (0.00%)	0 (0.00%) (0.00%)	3(42.86%) (30.00%)	0 (0.00%) (0.00%)	4 (57.14%) (40.00%)	0 (0.00%) (0.00%)	7 (100.00%) (11.67%)	
Sheet_metal	10 (50.00%) (100.00%)	0 (0.00%) (0.00%)	0 (0.00%) (0.00%)	0(0.00%) (0.00%)	0 (0.00%) (0.00%)	10 (50.00%) (100.00%)	20 (100.00%) (33.33%)	
s	0 (0.00%) (0.00%)	10(30.3%) (100.%)	7(21.21%) (70%)	10(30.30%) (100%)	6 (18.18%) (60%)	0 (0.00%) (0.00%)	33 (100.00%) (55.00%)	

Table 5.
Factors influencing malaria transmission in sites.

Characteristic	(Intercept)	Coefficient*	Odds ratio	Lower 95% CI limit	Upper 95% CI limit	P-value
Site distance	6.43243243	−0.05882353	0.9428731	0.9013153	0.9535306	0.04073
Number of people	2.00000000	0.08333333	1.086904	0.9512268	1.673181	0.196
House type	1.85624153	0.07423761	1.077063	0.9492531	1.638152	0.1822
ITN number	1.499946	1.000010	2.718282	2.518309	7.389241	0.02652
Child ≤5 years old	1.5000088	0.01287691	1.00296	1.00121	2.954372	0.6716
Fever ≤14 days	1.4759213	0.01174856	1.011818	1.010123	1.638152	0.4186

**Coefficients of the linear predictor of the resulting line of the logistic model. The exponential of these coefficients gives the odds ratio, the distance between the household and the breeding site; the number of people in the household; and house type.*

Table 6.
Determination of factors influencing anapheline density.

sunny stagnant surfaces, pools with erect vegetation, brackish water, etc. But *An. gambiae s.l.* preferentially uses residual pools of sunlit stagnant surfaces in several regions of Africa [24]. It is important to point out in the DRC with the advent of decentralization which increased the number of provinces from 11 to 26, a lot of modernization and urbanization work has been carried out in the new provinces to accommodate the provincial institutions.

Overall, correct urbanization reduces the risk of malaria transmission [1]. However, this urbanization has been anarchic in many provinces and has favored focal transmission of malaria, which results in a high disease burden [1, 4]. This anarchic urbanization is exacerbated by human activities which create temporary and artificial shelters favorable to the development of *An. gambaie sl* throughout the year [11, 12].

All urban areas of the DRC have almost the same ecology (large sunny space and the larval sites created by human activities). This ecology is favorable for the development of *An. gambiae s.l.* These results would reflect a low diversity observed. On the other hand, these results do not corroborate those of Rahm and Vermylen [15] and Sinka et al. [25], who found 61 species at the ecological scale of all the territories of the DRC.

2.3.2 Determination of entomological parameters

In general, the entomological indices of transmission are very high in the three capture sites. Despite high anopheline densities observed in Boende (Boende 2 health area) at 10 *An.*/house and in Mweka (Mweka health area) at 9 *An.*/house, compared to the Lisala site, no significant difference was observed. These highly observed densities can be justified by the poor quality of the habitat observed in these sites [26]. In addition, the absence of ITNs and the presence of larval sites also positively influenced anopheline density.

And we observed a high rate of *Anopheles* engorgement in the different households. The Boende site recorded more gorged *Anopheles* due to the absence of mosquito nets and a lot of shelter. There is a significant difference between distance from houses and larval sites. The houses of the Antenne site were very distant from the larval sites. Anopheline density was lower in houses located far from larval sites (protective effect).

The anopheline density of gorged *Anopheles* mosquitoes was twice as high in houses with more impregnated mosquito nets (poor quality of mosquito nets found).

The contraction on the effectiveness of ITNs is justified by the fact that ITNs were dilapidated and also the observed low durability [27]. In the Boende and Lisala sites, the ITNs' distribution campaign took place in 2016 (problem with the quality of ITNs found in households). The other two variables were not statistically significant.

It is observed that malaria transmission is intense in Mweka with a very high entomological HBR index of 19.8 bites/human/night and EIR index of 2.73 infectious bites/human/night. and This contrasts with the good coverage in ITNs of 90% recorded in 1 year after the mass distribution of ITNs. There is also a strong resistance of *An. gambiae s.l.* to Alphacypermethrin (61%) and Deltamethrin (56%). These observations corroborate those of Metelo et al. [28] in Bandundu-ville and Apinjoh et al. [29]. These observations require a study to evaluate the effectiveness of ITNs in the context of malaria endemicity and resistance of *An. gambiae s.l.* to insecticides.

Anopheles behaviors were more endophilic and endophagic in all collection sites. The aggressive cycle started early around 6 p.m. and peaked around 12 a.m. This activity remained intense all night with high rates of aggressiveness, infectivity and entomological inoculation rate in all sites. It emerges that these sentinel sites, which are located at different locations and climatic conditions, thus present the same condition of transmission of malaria and the same incidence.

2.3.3 Anopheles susceptibility profile of gambiae s.l. against common insecticides

For more than a decade, the NMCP has been carrying out mass distribution campaigns for ITNs in order to obtain wide coverage (≥80%) for effective protection of the vulnerable population [4]. The widespread use of ITNs must require regular monitoring of the sensitivity of wild *Anopheles* populations to the insecticides used in the fight for resistance management [30]. This is the subject of the creation of sentinel sites for monitoring malaria vector bionomics and resistance [4].

It emerges from our study that DDT was ineffective in all sites and no knockdown effect (Kdt_{50} and Kdt_{95}) was achieved. The populations of *An. gambiae s.l.* in all sites exhibited high resistance (11–19%). These results corroborate those of Basilua et al. [13], Watsenga et al. [9] and Metelo et al. [31]. This is justified by the fact that these sites were agricultural sites at the time and benefited from the use of pesticides.

Deltamethrin and Alphacypermethrin reached Kdt_{50} late almost everywhere, except in Nyakunde. Deltamethrin was less effective compared to Alphacypermethrin. Anyway, the two pyrethroids (Deltamethrin and Alphacypermethrin) were less effective and the wild populations of *An. gambiae s.l.* have been resistant to them. Curiously after pre-exposure of *An. gambiae s.l.* to PBO, the efficacy of these two pyrethroids was restored at all sites.

3. Conclusions

The transmission of malaria is intense in the sentinel sites of the NMCP and is located in the same epidemiological facies where the conditions of transmission of the disease and the incidence are identical. This situation is aggravated by noncompliance with ITN distribution cycles and poor durability. This transmission is ensured by the *An. gambiae s.l.* with high resistance statuses to pyrethroids (Deltamethrin and Alphacypermethrin). The ecological choice is necessary for a good representation.

In addition, this study will allow the development of mapping and will serve as a benchmark for future entomological assessments to improve malaria surveillance in the DRC.

Acknowledgements

Our sincere thanks to Prof. Dr. Jean-Jacques Muyembe, Director General of the National Institute of Biomedical Research, for his support. Thank you teams of entomologists from INRB and KPSK for their support. We are very grateful to Marianne Sinka for correcting the English grammar.

Conflict of interest

The authors declare no conflict of interest.

Author details

Emery Metelo[1,2,3]*, Josue Zanga[4], Doudou Batumbo[2], Bien-aimé Mandja[2], Hyacinthe Lukoki[1,3], Arsène Bokulu[1,3], Trèsor Iluku[1,4], Narcisse Basosila[3,5], Emile Manzambi[1], Fiacre Agossa[6] and Erick Mukomena[5,7]

1 Institut National de Recherche Biomédicale, Kinshasa, RD Congo

2 Faculté de Médecine, Université de Bandundu, Bandundu-Ville, RD Congo

3 Faculté de Sciences et Technologie, Université de Kinshasa, Kinshasa, RD Congo

4 Faculté de Médecine, Université de Kinshasa, Kinshasa, RD Congo

5 Hygiène et Prévention Programme National de Lutte contre le Paludisme, Ministère de la Santé Publique, RD, Congo

6 PMI VectorLink Project, Abt Associates, Rockville, MD, USA

7 Faculté de Médecine, Université de Lubumbashi, Lubumbashi, RD Congo

*Address all correspondence to: pathymetelo@gmail.com

IntechOpen

© 2024 The Author(s). Licensee IntechOpen. This chapter is distributed under the terms of the Creative Commons Attribution License (http://creativecommons.org/licenses/by/3.0), which permits unrestricted use, distribution, and reproduction in any medium, provided the original work is properly cited.

References

[1] WHO. World Malaria Report 2021. Geneva: World Health Organization; 2021

[2] OMS. Weekly epidemiological record Relevé épidémiologique hebdomadaire. Vol. 97. Genève: OMS; 2022. pp. 429-452. Available from: http://www.who.int/wer

[3] Ilombe G, Matangila JR, Lulebo A, et al. Malaria among children under 10 years in 4 endemic health areas in Kisantu health zone: Epidemiology and transmission. Malaria Journal. 2023;**22**:3

[4] PNLP_RDC. Plan national stratégique Paludisme en République Démocratique du Congo (RDC) 2021-2023. Kinshasa RD Congo: Programme National de Lutte contre le Paludisme; 2021-2023

[5] Emina JBO, Doctor HV, Yé Y. Profiling malaria infection among under-five children in the Democratic Republic of Congo. PLoS One. 2021;**16**(5):e0250550

[6] Bien-Aimé MM, Brembilla A, Handschumacher P, Bompangue D, Gonzalez J-P, Muyembe J-J, et al. Temporal and spatial dynamics of Monkeypox in Democratic Republic of Congo, 2000-2015. Eco Health. 2019;**16**(3):476-487. DOI: 10.1007/s10393-019-01435-1

[7] MICS. Institut national de statistique (INS) RDC. Enquête par grappe à indicateurs multiples, 2017-2018. Kinshasa, République Démocratique du Congo: Rapport de résultats de l'enquête; 2019

[8] Yang GG, Kim D, Pham A, Paul CJ. A meta-regression analysis of the effectiveness of mosquito nets for malaria control: The value of long-lasting insecticide nets. International Journal of Environmental Research and Public Health. 2018;**15**(3):546. DOI: 10.3390/ijerph15030546

[9] Watsenga F, Riveron JM, Irving H, Irish SR. High plasmodium infection rate and reduced BeD net efficacy in multiple insecticide-resistant malaria vectors in Kinshasa, Democratic Republic of Congo. The Journal of Infectious Diseases. 2018;**217**(2):320-328

[10] PNLP-RDC. Revue a mi-parcours du plan strategique national 2016-2020: Defis et perspectives. Programme de lutte contre le paludisme. Kinshasa RD Congo: PNLP-RDC; 2018

[11] Mala Albert O, Irungu LW, Shililu JI, Muturi EJ, Mbogo CC, Njagi JK, et al. Dry season ecology of *Anopheles gambiae* complex mosquitoes at larval habitats in two traditionally semi-arid villages in Baringo, Kenya. Parasites & Vectors. 2011;**4**:25

[12] Hinne Isaac A, Attah SK, Mensah BA, Forson AO, Afrane YA. Larval habitat diversity and Anopheles mosquito species distribution in different ecological zones in Ghana. Parasites and Vectors. 2021;**14**:193. DOI: 10.1186/s13071-021-04701-w

[13] Basilua Kanza JP, El Fahime E, Alaoui S, Essassi EM, Brooke B, Nkebolo Malafu A, et al. Pyrethroid, DDT and malathion resistance in the malaria vector *Anopheles gambiae* from the Democratic Republic of Congo. Transactions of the Royal Society of Tropical Medicine and Hygiene. 2013;**107**(1):8-14

[14] Metelo E, Kaounga MMGI, Zanga J, Mbuku GB, et al. Insecticide susceptibility of *Anopheles gambiae* s.l

and identification of some resistance mechanisms in Kwilu Province in the Democratic Republic of Congo. Pan African Medical Journal. 2020;**37**:79

[15] Rahm U, Vermylen M. Repertoire et repartition des Anopheles de la Republique Democratique du Congo. Estratto dalla Rivisita di Malariologia. 1966;**65**:1-3

[16] Kwi P, Ewane E, Moyeh M, Tangi L, Ntui V, Zeukeng F, et al. Diversity and behavioral activity of anopheles mosquitoes on the slopes of Mount Cameroon. Parasites & Vectors. 2022;**15**:344. DOI: 10.1186/s13071-022-05472-8

[17] Pinto J, Williams J. Manuel de Formation à l'Entomologie du Paludisme à l'intention des techniciens en entomologie et lutte anti-vectorielle. U.S.A. Research Triangle Park: RTI International; 2012

[18] WHO. Tests Procedures for Insecticide Resistance Monitoring in Malaria Vector Mosquitoes. Vol. 2. Geneva: WHO; 2016. p. 55

[19] Gnanguenon V, Renaud G, Agossa F, Razaki O, Frédéric O, Roseric A, et al. Transmission patterns of plasmodium falciparum by *Anopheles gambiae* in Benin. Malaria Journal. 2014;**13**:444, Available from: http://www.malariajournal.com/content/13/1/444

[20] Tchuinkam T, Simard F, Lélé-Defo E, Téné-Fossog B, al. RBeiseoarncho armticleics of Anopheline species and malaria transmission dynamics along an altitudinal transect in Western Cameroon. BMC Infectious Diseases. 2010;**10**:119. Available from: http://www.biomedcentral.com/1471-2334/10/119

[21] Gillies MT, De Meillon B. The Anophelinae of Africa south of the Sahara (Ethiopian zoogeographical region). Publication of the South of African institute for Medical Research, Johannesburg. 1968;**2**(54):343

[22] Coetzee M. Key to the females of Afrotropical anopheles mosquitoes (Diptera: Culicidae). Malaria Journal. 2020;**19**:70. DOI: 10.1186/s12936-020-3144-9

[23] Mouchet J, Carnavale P, Coosemans M, Julvez J, Richard-Lenoble D, Sircoulon J. Biodiversite du paludisme dans le monde. Vol. 1. Eurotest Paris: Ed John Libbey; 2004. pp. 12-96

[24] Edillo FE, Touré YT, Lanzaro GC, Dolo G, Taylor CE. Survivorship and distribution of immature *Anopheles gambiae* s.l. (Diptera: Culicidae) in Banambani Village, Mali. Journal of Medical Entomology. 2004;**41**:333-339

[25] Marianne S, Davide Z, Yunpeng L, Ivan K, Dickson M, Japhet K, et al. Hum bug–an acoustic mosquito monitoring tool for use on budget smartphones. Ecology and Evolution. 2021;**12**:1848-1859

[26] Dlamini N, Hsiang MS, Ntshalintshali N, Pindolia D, Allen R, Nhlabathi N, et al. Low-quality housing is associated with increased risk of malaria infection: A National Population-Based Study from the low transmission setting of Swaziland. Open Forum Infectious Diseases. 2017;**4**(2):ofx071

[27] Mansiangi P, Umesumbu S, Etewa I, Zandibeni J, Bafwa N, Blaufuss S, et al. Comparing the durability of the longlasting insecticidal nets DawaPlus ® 2.0 and DuraNet© in northwest Democratic Republic of Congo. Malaria Journal. 2020;**19**:189

[28] Metelo E, Zanga J, Nsabatien V, Mbala A, Ngamukie S, Agossa F, et al.

Effect of the mass distribution of ITNs in an endemic area with a high entomological index, the case of Bandundu-City, Kwilu, DRC [internet]. In: Mosquito Research - Recent Advances in Pathogen Interactions, Immunity, and Vector Control Strategies. London, UK: IntechOpen; 2023

[29] Apinjoh TO, Anchang-Kimbi JK, Mugri RN, Tangoh DA, Nyingchu RV, Chi HF, et al. The effect of insecticide treated nets (ITNs) on plasmodium falciparum infection in rural and semi-urban communities in the south west region of Cameroon. PLoS One. 2015;**10**(2):e0116300. DOI: 10.1371/journal.pone.0116300

[30] PNLP_RDC. Plan national de gestion de la résistance des vecteurs du Paludisme aux insecticides en République Démocratique du Congo (RDC) 2022-2024. Kinshasa RD Congo: Programme National de Lutte contre le Paludisme; 2022

[31] Metelo E, Zanga J, Binene G, Mvuama N, Ngamukie S, Nkey J, et al. The effect of a mass distribution of insecticide-treated nets on insecticide resistance and entomological inoculation rates of *Anopheles gambiae* s.l. in Bandundu City, Democratic Republic of Congo. The Pan African Medical Journal. 2021;**40**:118

Section 3

Malaria Diagnosis

Chapter 6

Advanced Techniques and Unusual Samples for Malaria Diagnosis

Ismail Muhammad, Micah Pukuma Sale and Tanko Mahmoud Mohammed

Abstract

Successful malaria control, treatment, and prevention depends on successful diagnosis using appropriate equipment with high sensitivity and specificity. In most tropical countries where the disease is endemic, malaria diagnosis is still based on the conventional techniques (Microscopy and RDT) which have so many shortcomings, hence the need to switch to the most advanced diagnostic technique for better results. In this review, several serological and molecular malaria diagnostic techniques like Polymerase Chain Reaction (PCR), Flow cytometry, Loop-mediated Isothermal Amplification (LAMP), Indirect Immunofluorescence, Enzyme-Linked Immunosorbent Assay (ELISA), Radioimmunoassay (RIA), Quantitative Buffy Coat (QBC) and Laser Desorption Mass Spectrometry (LDMS) were systematically discussed in simple and direct language for easier understanding of the principle involved in each case scenario. In addition, some unusual samples for malaria diagnosis like Urine and saliva were also discussed.

Keywords: diagnosis, polymerase chain reaction, quantitative Buffy coat, *plasmodium falciparum*, flow cytometry, saliva

1. Introduction

1.1 Malaria diagnoses

Successful prevention, treatment, and eradication of malaria infection heavily depend on the successful diagnosis, as a result, the Word Health Organisation (WHO) stresses the need for effective, reliable, and dependable diagnosis and confirmation before any form of intervention [1, 2], thus, discourages any form of intervention before laboratory diagnosis and confirmation [3, 4]. This is because, clinical diagnosis alone is not enough to confirm the presence or absence of malaria infection [5], as the clinical signs and symptoms of the disease mimic many other tropical diseases [6], which could be hardly differentiated from malaria infection [7, 8].

Malaria diagnosis usually involves identifying the parasite, or parasite's products (antigens) in the blood of the subjects. In most tropical parts of the globe, except for some rare and special cases, malaria diagnosis is based on conventional techniques, like Microscopy [9] which is regarded as the gold standard technique [10] and Rapid

Diagnostic Technique (RDT) [11] using either venous blood or hand prick blood as the case may be. To some extent, conventional diagnostic techniques like RDTs are easy to perform as they require less training and expertise, and are cost-effective, with an appreciable level of Sensitivity and Specificity. With all these advantages, conventional diagnostic techniques have some limitations and challenges that in some cases underscore their actual performance. Some of these limitations include detecting sequestered parasites (*Plasmodium* species) in tissues like the placenta and liver. In addition, they are less reliable when the level of parasitaemia is very low, as the techniques are not able to detect the presence of the parasite below a certain threshold. These and so many other factors led to either false positive or false negative results [12], and the accumulation of such diagnostic results in a population seriously affects the prevention, control, treatment and elimination of malaria infection generally. This is because such diagnostic result, especially false negative always ensures the presence of a reservoir host of malaria infection in a given population, as the infected individuals may go unnoticed and untreated [13].

Advanced malaria diagnostic techniques have the potential to overcome all these shortcomings observed in conventional techniques [14]. Unlike the conventional techniques, they are quite expensive and require special training and expertise, but they produce the much-needed results with a high level of sensitivity and specificity (Accuracy) [15], especially when performed under appropriate and conducive laboratory conditions and also by applying the principles of quality control and quality assurance in handling and treating all samples for malaria diagnosis. To that effect, advanced diagnostic techniques are very much needed especially in countries and places where malaria infection is still endemic (Sub-Sahran Africa), as the techniques always ensure the real confirmation of the deadly parasites (*Plasmodium*). Therefore, when appropriate treatment is applied to the confirmed positive subjects, this automatically breaks the chain of transmission, which may lead to successful elimination of the disease.

Nevertheless, conventional malaria diagnostic techniques are still very relevant, especially in underdeveloped and developing tropical countries where electricity which is one of the basic requirements for almost all the advanced techniques is still a topical issue. In addition, some of the advanced diagnostic techniques are automatically not suitable for routine laboratory diagnosis, instead, they only serve as confirmatory or screening of blood donors during blood transfusion. For better results, therefore, both conventional and advanced malaria diagnostic techniques should be married together. In this regard, conventional techniques should not be completely ignored at the expense of advanced Techniques. Nevertheless, the selection and adoption of a given diagnostic technique heavily depend on the peculiarities of the area and its inhabitants which include; level of endemicity, geographical accessibility, social and economic characteristics, underlying health infrastructure, available diagnostic tools and prevalence and type of drug resistance [16].

Given the foregoing discourse, this paper aims to systematically review the state of knowledge on different advanced malaria diagnostic techniques like Polymerase Chain Reaction (PCR), Flow cytometry, Loop-mediated Isothermal Amplification (LAMP), Indirect Immunofluorescence, Enzyme-Linked Immunosorbent Assay (ELISA), Radioimmunoassay (RIA), Quantitative Buffy Coat (QBC) and Laser Desorption Mass Spectrometry which will be discussed in simple and direct language for easier understanding and comprehending. In addition, some unusual samples for malaria diagnosis like Urine and saliva will also be looked at in this review.

2. Quantitative buffy coat

The quantitative Buffy Coat Technique is an advanced form of conventional microscopy, unlike conventional microscopy, it is only a qualitative screening technique not quantitative [17]. This diagnostic technique is by far more sensitive (almost 8 times more sensitive) than conventional microscopy [18, 19].

This technique is applied for malaria diagnosis based on: centrifugation, density gradient of infected erythrocytes and fluorescence. The technique is good enough to detect the presence of malaria parasites as low as 5 parasites per μL of blood sample [20–22]. The QBC technique is performed with the aid of a capillary tube coated with a fluorescence dye, usually, an acridine orange stain is used. This stain when excited to a frequency of 460 nm allows the detection of the parasite at a lower frequency [23].

Briefly, about 3–5 μl of blood is collected into the tube containing anticoagulant and centrifuge at 1200 g for 5 minute, this makes the blood sample separated and differentiated into different components (Plasma, Platelets, Moncyte/Lymphocyte, Red blood cells etc.) inform of layers based on their density gradient and also even the parasites are separated into different layers based on their developmental stages [24]. For example, gametocytes being lighter than schizont, mature trophozoite and ring form are found at the top layer, while ring form being the heaviest of all are found at the extreme lower part of the tube with red blood cells. The stain (acridine orange) contained in the tube stains the genetic material (DNA and RNA) and cytoplasm of the *Plasmodium* parasite. When observed under blue-violet light through a microscope (fluorescent microscope) the nucleus fluoresces bright green while the cytoplasm fluoresces yellow-green, thus revealing the morphological features of the *Plasmodium* parasite [19].

Some major drawbacks of this technique are; the expensiveness of the technique, very difficult in determining *Plasmodium* species at the ring form stage, and very easy in arriving at false positive results/conclusions due to the presence of artefacts such as cell debris [25].

3. Serological technique for malaria diagnosis

In common parlance, serology is the scientific study of serum and other body fluids. Technically, different serological techniques are now available and applied for the diagnosis of several parasitic and infectious diseases. All serological techniques act on the same principle, which is an antigen-antibody reaction [26]. The simple secret behind this technique is that in all foreign bodies (parasites or any infectious agent) whenever they invade a system, the system or body automatically produces antibodies in response to that [27] while the foreign body produces antigens. For example in the case of *Plasmodium falciparum* malaria, antigens such as Merozoite Surface Protein 2 (MSP-2), Apical Membrane Antigen 1(APM-1), and Erythrocyte Binding Antigen 175 (EBA-175) [28], Histidine Rich Protein 2 (HRP-2) (produced only by *Plasmodium falciparum*) Plasmodium Lactate Dehyrogenase (pLDH) (produced by the all four species) which are usually found in serum of the infected individuals [29]. Therefore, in serological diagnostic techniques for malaria parasites, such specific antigens produced by the asexual stage of *Plasmodium* species are the main target in the serum or plasma of the suspected individuals.

Nevertheless, one important point worth mentioning here is that serological techniques for malaria diagnosis, generally are not highly recommended and suitable for routine diagnosis of malaria infection [30]. This is because all serological techniques are based on antibodies generated or produced after initial infection with a given *Plasmodium* species, and this may take a minimum period of 2 weeks [31], and it may persist in either serum or plasma for about 3–6 months. Therefore, serological-techniques are more suitable and recommended in non-endemic areas where the results revealed by other diagnostic technique is doubtful, and for determining prior exposure to the malaria parasite, epidemiological investigations or screening blood donor [32, 33], to prevent transfusion-induced malaria especially when level of parasitaemia is too low to be diagnosed by conventional techniques like microscopy.

3.1 Immunofluorescence antibody testing for malaria diagnosis

3.1.1 Indirect immunofluorescence

In this, a known antigen of *Plasmodium* species is placed onto a grease-free glass slide, smeared and allowed to air-dry, after which it is then fixed with acetone for 1–2 minute. After which, a serum which is expectedly to contain *Plasmodium* species antibody is added onto the smeared slide. Therefore, the antigen-antibody complex generated can then be detected by adding anti-human immunoglobulin (IgG) labelled with a fluorescein Isothiocynate (FIT), this binds to the antibody in the serum and when observed under a fluorescence microscope with the aid UV light, a fluorescence is observed, which confirm a positive sample.

Of all the available serological techniques, the immunofluorescence Antibody Technique (IFA) is considered the "Gold Standard Technique" due to its high level of Sensitivity and Specificity compared to other serological techniques, very easy to perform and reproducible technique, to some extent provides good evidence of recent infection [34]. However, it is time-consuming and subjective, especially with a serum that has low antibody titre. The basic principle of this technique, like all other serological techniques is based on antigen-antibody reactions. Normally, two weeks after initial infection with any of the *Plasmodium* species, antibodies are generated, which persist in the blood for about 2–3 months even after parasite clearance (Treatment) [35]. In this technique, the ratio of IgG to IgM serves as the measure and determinant factor for the positivity of a given sample and also for identifying recent infection, which is vital for epidemiological studies and also one peculiar advantage of the technique [36]. Therefore, in this, when the titre value (IgG: IgM) is greater than 1:20 is regarded as POSITIVE, while a titre value less than 1:20 is regarded as a UNCONFIRMED malaria sample and a sample with a titre value greater than 1:200 is regarded as RECENT INFECTION [35].

3.2 Enzyme-linked immunosorbent assay

Unlike the immunofluorescence Antibody Technique which is time-consuming, ELISA has been considered to be a fast, Sensitive and specific method for the detection of malaria parasites [37]. It works by detecting the presence of different antibodies of *Plasmodium species*. It is usually used to screen blood donors before transfusion [38] to prevent possible transmission of malaria parasites to the patients. There are different commercially prepared ELISA kits, for example, Trinity Biotech, cellabs, DiaPro, newbio, Novatec [39], etc. The practical application and utilisation of each of the kits strictly depends on the recommendation and description of the protocol/procedure by the manufacturers of the kit. Nevertheless, all ELISA kits work on the same basic principle and contain the same components, which include the following: Positive control, Negative Control, Conjugate, Conjugate dilution, Buffer, Substrate, Wash, Stop and Microplate (comprised of 96 wells). Malaria ELISA kit uses four recombinants antigens in a sandwich test to detect IgG, IgM and IgA of either *Plasmodium falcifarum, P. vivix, P. malariae, P.ovale* during all stages of malaria infection, but most attention is on IgG and IgM [40].

The basic general principle of ELISA is as follows; Coated microplate with specific antigens binds to the corresponding antibodies of the sample. All unreacted material in the sample, which is Horseradish peroxide are removed, followed by the addition of a conjugate [41]. The conjugate binds to the captured antibodies, this is followed by the second wash to remove all unreacted conjugate. The pure antigen-antibody complex generated is visualised by adding a substrate (Tetramethyl Benzidine), thereby forming a product which is green in colour. The intensity of the colour is always proportional to the amount of specific antibodies present in the test sample. Sulphuric acid (a stop) is added to completely stop the reaction. This gives rise to a yellow colouration of the reaction. Finally, absorbance at 450 nm is read using an ELISA reader.

The following steps summarise the procedural protocol of Enzyme-linked Immunosorbent Assay. Briefly, dispense 50 μL of the sample (serum or plasma) into a coated well of the well of the plate and shake the loaded plate for 30 seconds using a plate shaker. Use the wash buffer to wash five times, between each wash cycle soak for 30 seconds, after which remove the excess liquid. To each well containing the test sample add 50 μL of the already diluted conjugate and incubate for 30 minutes at 37° C, after which make a second (five times) wash and soak again, then also remove the excess liquid. This is followed by the addition of 50 μL of substrate/Chromogene mixture and incubation at room temperature for 30 minutes, after which add 50 μL of stop (Sulphuric acid) to each well. This makes the colour change from blue to yellow, and then finally reads the absorbance of each sample in an ELISA reader at 450 nm.

3.2.1 Validation of the test technique

The validity of the ELISA test heavily depends on meeting the following requirement, and failure to meet the requirement, may consider the test invalid and need to be repeated.

a. absorbance of substrate blank = < 0.1

b. absorbance of Negative control = 0.200 < Cut-off

c. absorbance of Cut-off = 0.15–1.3

d. absorbance of positive control > Cut-off

3.2.2 Cut-off point determination

This can determine by taking the average of the negative control values and adding 0.100 which is

$$\frac{\text{Negative Control 1} + \text{Negative Control 2} + \text{Negative Control 3}}{3} \tag{1}$$

3.2.3 Result interpretation

Samples with A_{450} value above the cut-off value are considered as POSITIVE, on the other hand, if the A_{450} is less than the cut-off value, the result is regarded as NEGATIVE.

NB: For all negative samples ($A_{450} <$ cut-off), if the difference is not that significant, such samples should be interpreted with extra care. Therefore, such samples should be re-tested again.

3.3 Radioimmunoassay

In the 1950s, two New York Scientists Rosalan Yalow and Solomon Berson invented the technique of Radioimmunoassay. It is a serological diagnostic technique that is regarded as highly sensitive with also high level of specificity. The technique has a very good ability to detect the presence of antigen/protein and hormones in a clinical sample as low as one part in a billion (Nanogram of antigen in a serum). Its high level of sensitivity is attributed to the use of Radionuclides while the specificity is solely associated with the immunochemical reaction, hence the name Radioimmunoassay.

The basic principle on which RIA operates, in addition to antigen-antibody reaction which is common to all other serological techniques, also involves a competitive binding to antibodies between labelled and unlabelled antigens to form antigen-antibody complexes. After initial infection with *Plasmodium* species, antigens are produced, and in return the B-lymphocytes secrete antibodies. In the RIA, the serum containing the antibodies is collected and treated with radioactive antigens followed by non-radioactive antigens. Two main reactions take place in the process of RIA, as shown in the equations below; first, a reaction between the unlabelled antigen (*Plasmodium* antigen to be determined in serum) and the antibody generated. Second reaction is the reaction between a labelled antigen and the same antibody, thus creating a competition between labelled and unlabelled antigens, but this competition always favours the labelled antigen, as it always over the unlabelled antigen.

$$\text{Unlabelled antigen (Ag)} + \textit{Plasmodium} \text{ antibody (Ab)} =\!=' \text{UAg—Ab complex} \ldots \ldots .(\text{Rxn } 1)$$

$$\text{Labelled antigen (Ag}^*) + \textit{Plasmodium} \text{ antibody (Ab)} =\!=' \text{UAg}^*\text{—Ab complex} \ldots \ldots .(\text{Rxn } 2)$$

Or

$$\text{Unlabelled antigen (Ag)} + \textit{Plasmodium} \text{ antibody (Ab)} =\!=' \text{UAg—Ab complex} \ldots \ldots .(\text{Rxn } 1)$$

$$+$$

$$\text{Labelled antigen (Ag}^*)$$

$$\downarrow$$

$$\text{Ag}^*\text{—Ab complex} \ldots \ldots .(\text{Rxn } 2)$$

Therefore, the amount of the *Plasmodium* species antigens will be determined by the amount of radioactivity. Therefore, one good aspect of RIA is that it can be applied for both qualitative and quantitative determination of antigens without the use of bioassays.

4. Molecular techniques

4.1 Polymerase chain reaction

Polymerase Chain Reaction is an advanced molecular technique that has been known to be used in the diagnosis of genetic and infectious diseases including malaria, the technique is usually applied for the confirmation of different *Plasmodium* species in a given sample [42], especially when the outcomes of other conventional technique (e.g Microscopy and or RDTs) indicate negative results [43] and is more sensitive compared other conventional techniques [44], especially when the parasitaemia level is very low [45]. Some studies have shown that PCR has recorded a sensitivity and specificity of 100% each by detecting 1–3 *Plasmodium* parasite/μL of blood samples and it also has a good ability to detect mixed infection [46]. PCR like other advanced malaria diagnostic techniques is not usually adopted as a routine technique as it uses very expensive reagent/kit (DNA extraction kit) and other equipment (for example thermocycler) [47] and above all, the whole process starts from DNA extraction, DNA amplification and running of the gels all require steady electricity which is still lacking in most tropical countries where the malaria infection is still endemic [48], as it can hardly be effectively adopted in resource-poor endemic countries [49]. PCR-based diagnosis for malaria infection targets the subunit Ribosomal RNA gene (18 s-rRNA) for the detection of different *Plasmodium* species [50]. This is because the gene is universally present in all *Plasmodia* species, coupled with the fact that it has a very strong inter and intra-specie conserved region and is always readily available in large quantities [51].

Apart from the conventional PCR-based assay, there are other different forms of PCR which are purposely designed to overcome the shortcomings of other diagnostic techniques, these include Nested PCR, Quantitative PCR (qPCR) and Multiplex PCR [52, 53] and all PCR work on the same basic principle, but one of the main shortcomings of the technique is that it requires much longer time compared to microscopy and RDTs.

Nested PCR involves primary (first) and secondary (second) PCR, in which universal primers are used for the amplification of the conserved sequence of the small subunit rRNA genes from the *Plasmodium species,* while the secondary PCR is carried out with primers that are specific to each *Plasmodium* species [54]. Other target sequences used by the nested PCR include the Merozoite surface antigen (MSA) gene and Erythrocyte binding antigen (EBA-175) [55]. In this, the amplicons (PCR products) generated from the primary PCR serve as a DNA template for the secondary PCR. Therefore, by this, two rounds of amplification are generated, which makes it very possible for a single genome of a given *Plasmodium* species to be detected and reproduce in large quantities. Two important factors that determine the sensitivity and success of whole processes are the quantity and purity of the starting material which is the DNA template.

Quantitative PCR allows the detection and quantification of the target DNA through the use of fluorophore probes. This method has a detection limit of 0.02 p/μl for genus-level identification, and 1.22 parasite/μl for *P. falciparum* detection, while multiplex PCR, as the name implies, can detect multiple *Plasmodium* species, with a detection limit of 0.2–5parasite/μl of the suspected sample [56].

4.2 Loop-mediated isothermal amplification

The technique, which was developed 23 years back [57], unlike other molecular techniques like PCR, is simple, less time-consuming, requires less sophisticated equipment and can be adopted even in a field with a high level of accuracy [58]. It has a very good ability to detect positive malaria samples even at a very low level of parasitaemia (1–2 parasite/μL of blood) this serves as an additional advantage over conventional microscopy which cannot detect the infection when the parasite density is very low. Missing such patients in a population always ensures the presence of a reservoir host. LAMP can be used to detect the presence of all four *Plasmodia* species in a suspected sample by determining the presence of the parasite's DNA in a single Isothermal step in the presence of an enzyme (*Bacillus stearothermophilus* Polymerase) [59] that can separate the double-stranded DNA without temperature denaturation and four to six specific primers [60].

For malaria parasite, the first set of primers is designed to target six to eight sites along the 18S ribosomal RNA gene (18SrRNA) of the genus *Plasmodium*, unlike PCR at a single temperature (60–65°C) [61], this increases the high specificity of the technique, while other primers target mitochondrial DNA, thus, improving the sensitivity of the technique. The auto-cycling strand-displacement DNA generates a large amount of stem-loop DNA copies (roughly 109) of different sizes through an amplification process in less than an hour [62]. This is produced together with insoluble magnesium pyrophosphate (a by-product of DNA synthesis) which is normally generated in proportion to the amplified gene [63].

The insoluble magnesium pyrophosphate produced in the reaction looks turbid and can be seen with the naked eye, this can be used to interpret the LAMP result. Nevertheless, sometimes the visualisation of magnesium pyrophosphate precipitate is a little bit difficult, especially when the DNA concentration is relatively low. A sample is considered to be positive or negative if an obvious increase in the turbidity is observed by the naked eye compared to the negative control, in addition, a LAMP test/result is considered valid if the turbidity is present in the positive control but completely absent in the negative control [64]. The result also can be interpreted by the use of ultraviolet (UV) fluorescent in the presence of an indicator such as Calcein. On the other hand, real-time detection of results is possible using a Loop real-time turbidimeter. In addition, LAMP results can be interpreted using either colorimetic and fluorescent or Lateral flow detection [65]. Detailed procedures and protocol of LAMP technique for malaria diagnosis heavily depend on the specific type of kit used, as there are different commercially available LAMP kits and each with its specifications, for example, Illumigene (Alethia), malaria LAMP, and Loopamp malaria amplification kit [66]. One of the short-comings of this technique it is qualitative, not quantitative, but has a very good sensitivity similar to other sensitive molecular techniques like PCR [67].

4.3 Laser desorption mass spectrometry

Laser Desorption Mass Spectrometry for malaria diagnosis depends on the detection of heme from hemezoin, which is an insoluble microcrystal generated during haemoglobin digestion by the *Plasmodium* parasite, thus, this serves as a biomarker for malaria infection. The heme produced has a good potential of absorbing ultraviolet laser [68], as a result, it is also called malarial pigment [69]. LDMS is reported to have a very good sensitivity of 52% and specificity of 92% but the technique is not suitable in places where malaria infection is endemic and is not recommended for routine malaria diagnosis as the technique is quite expensive [70]. The detection limit of this technique is 10 parasites/µl of culture and 100 parasites/µl of the blood sample.

Unlike PCR and other molecular techniques, LDMS does not require sophisticated equipment or apparatus, instead only metal slides, sample collection bottles, distilled water and aliquot are required [71]. The LDMS technique is quite simple, straightforward and very fast to produce results (in fact in less than 1 minute), it only involves diluting the collected/suspected blood sample with the appropriate amount of buffer (Phosphate Buffer Saline) and placing it onto a metal slide and allow to air-dry, after which the prepared slide is inserted into a mass spectrometer for sample analysis. Heme-specific ions in RBCs are desorbed from the probe and analysed by their mass/charge ratio, generating a parasite-specific mass spectral signature [72].

4.4 Flow cytometry

For long, flow cytometry using scattering and fluorescent detection methods has been in use for many years as a fundamental instrument for disease diagnosis [73]. For malaria diagnosis, this technique, like Laser Desorption Mass Spectrometry depends on the detection and quantification of heme using a special machine called flow cytometer and also works on the principle of flow cytometry, hence, the name of the technique. This is a haematology analyser that is used for the presumptive diagnosis of malaria and other haematological parameters of the sample [74]. Different flow cytometric methods are used to determine the presence of the infection and also quantify the level of parasitaemia [75]. Flow cytometry is a measurement of characteristic single cells (cyto) suspended in a flowing saline stream, and is the only technique capable of rapidly identifying cells and parasites from large samples. It relies on scattering or fluorescence measurements that are made while the cells or particles pass through a capillary flow cell [76]. Flow cytometry work on three basic coordinated component, which include; fluidics, optical, and electronic systems [77]. Some of the disadvantages of this technique are its low sensitivity compared to other techniques and it also requires specialised equipment [78]. Therefore, this technique is not highly recommended for routine malaria diagnosis, especially in sub-Saharan Africa where the disease is highly endemic area.

5. Unusual samples for malaria diagnosis

Venus or hand prick blood are the well-known samples for malaria diagnosis in most laboratories in the endemic countries, as it is always readily much available except for some special cases/reasons. Most of the time, the blood serves as the preferred sample [79] as the parasite lives intra-cellularly, therefore this allows physical examination of the parasite (*Plasmodium*), its developmental stages and its other morphological features under a microscope.

Nevertheless, in some cases, the blood sample may not be easily and readily available due to some factors/reasons which include customs and natural beliefs, creed and religious beliefs [80], and fear of pricking or bleeding using a lancet or needle. In addition sometimes the parasite density in the peripheral blood tends to fluctuate, this is normally due to the sequestration of the parasites in tissues and other vital organs like the brain, spleen etc. [81]. Therefore to overcome all these and always make samples readily available for malaria diagnosis, the parasite's products (antigen for example Histidine Rich Protein-2, Plasmodium Lactate Dehydrogenase (pLDH)) can also be found in other body fluids and products like Urine [82] Saliva, Faeces and hair [83]. Apart from this, several abnormalities in urine like haematuria (possibly due to massive destruction of infected RBC by the parasite, thus leading to excretion of blood and even haemoglobin together with urine) and proteinuria have been attributed to malaria infection [84, 85]. Therefore, any of these (Urine, Saliva, faeces and Hair) samples can serve as a very good alternative sample for malaria diagnosis. The use of any of these non-invasive samples drastically reduces or eliminates the risk of infection to both the screener and the patient [86].

5.1 Urine

Urine Malaria Test (UMT) involves the determination of the presence of the parasite's antigen (Histidine Rich Protein-2 (HRP-2)) in a given suspected urine sample, this is because the antigen is water-soluble protein, and therefore it can be found in the urine [87]. In addition, urine is an ultra-filtrate of blood, it can be effectively used instead of blood for malaria diagnosis [88]. Like with the blood, there is a Urine-based RDT/Kit for malaria diagnosis, the detailed principle and protocol of the Urine-based RDT was explained in the work of [89]. In addition, DNA of the *Plasmodium* can also be recovered from the urine sample of the infected individuals, therefore, PCR can be employed to amplify the parasite's (*Plasmodium*) DNA from the urine sample [90]. The urine-Malaria Test technique has many additional advantages compared to the conventional blood-based RDT techniques, which include a lack of difficulties (searching for veins, pain during pricking and or bleeding) in obtaining a sample, also the process is non-invasive, thus eliminating the risk of infection and like blood- based RDT techniques is a very simple, easy technique and it requires less time compared to microscopy and other advanced molecular techniques [91].

5.2 Saliva

Saliva is regarded as a less invasive sample for malaria diagnosis, it contains markers such as antigen, DNA, and sequence of 16S RNA that are normally used as the best target for saliva-based RDT kits. Therefore, the presence of these in the saliva provided very good evidence of obtaining products (DNA and or Proteins) in the saliva of malaria-infected individuals [92]. Having saliva as a sample for malaria diagnosis offers many advantages over the conventional blood sample, these include; ease of collection, transportation and storage [93]. Therefore, like in other samples (blood and urine) the parasite's products can be detected using already known molecular techniques like PCR, nested PCR, qPCR etc.

Author details

Ismail Muhammad[1*], Micah Pukuma Sale[2] and Tanko Mahmoud Mohammed[3]

1 Department of Zoology, Gombe State University, Gombe, Nigeria

2 Department of Zoology, Modibbo Adama University, Yola, Nigeria

3 Department of Biomedical and Pharmaceutical Technology, Federal Polytechnic Mubi, Yola, Nigeria

*Address all correspondence to: muhammadismail5609@gsu.edu.ng

IntechOpen

© 2023 The Author(s). Licensee IntechOpen. This chapter is distributed under the terms of the Creative Commons Attribution License (http://creativecommons.org/licenses/by/3.0), which permits unrestricted use, distribution, and reproduction in any medium, provided the original work is properly cited.

References

[1] Aigbiremo M, Cheryl E, Ndiaye T, Sadikh A, Ndiaye D, Amambua-ngwa A. International journal of infectious diseases comparative analysis of four malaria diagnostic tools and implications for malaria treatment in southwestern Nigeria. International Journal of Infectious Diseases. 2021;**2021**(108): 377-381. DOI: 10.1016/j.ijid.2021.05.049

[2] Wellington NE, Oyibo A, Ntadom G, Oladosu OO, Kaitlin Rainwater-Loveth WO, Okpokoro E, et al. Cross Multicenter pivotal clinical trial of urine malaria test for rapid diagnosis of. Journal of Clinical Microbiology. 2017;**55**: 253-263

[3] Tagbor H, Bruce J, Browne E, Greenwood B, Chandramohan D. Performance of the OptiMAL ® dipstick in the diagnosis of malaria infection in pregnancy. Therapeutics and Clinical Risk Management. 2008;**4**(3): 631-636

[4] Maturana CR et al. Advances and challenges in automated malaria diagnosis using digital microscopy imaging with artificial intelligence tools : A review. Frontiers in Microbiology. 2022;**13**(1006659):1-17. DOI: 10.3389/fmicb.2022.1006659

[5] Mukry SN, Saud M, Sufaida G, Shaikh K, Naz A, Shamsi TS. Laboratory diagnosis of malaria: Comparison of manual and automated diagnostic tests. Canadian Journal of Infectious Diseases and Medical Microbiology. 2017;**2017** (Article ID 9286392):1-7

[6] Oladosu OO, Adedokun Victoria A, Akinkunle VA, Wellington O. Performance evaluation of malaria HRP-2 rapid diagnostic test among febrile patients with malaria in Iwo, Osun state, Nigeria. International Journal of Tropical Disease. 2021;**4**(1):1-9. DOI: 10.23937/2643-461X/1710046

[7] Calderaro A et al. Malaria diagnosis in non-endemic settings: The European experience in the last 22 years. Microorganisms. 2021;**9**(2265):1-25. DOI: 10.3390/microorganisms9112265

[8] Ojurongbe O et al. Assessment of clinical diagnosis , microscopy , rapid diagnostic tests , and polymerase chain reaction in the diagnosis of plasmodium falciparum in Nigeria. Malaria Research Treatment. 2013;**2013**(Article ID 308069):5-10

[9] Paul R, Bera SS, Nongrum S. A review of advance techniques in diagnosis of malaria. International Journal of Current Microbiology and Applied Science. 2016; **5**(11):631-636

[10] Yang D et al. A portable image-based cytometer for rapid malaria detection and quantification. PLoS One. 2017; **12**(6):1-18

[11] Mogeni P et al. Detecting malaria hotspots: A comparison of rapid diagnostic test, microscopy, and polymerase chain reaction. The Journal of Infectious Diseases. 2017;**216**: 1091-1098. DOI: 10.1093/infdis/jix321

[12] Yatsushiro S et al. Application of a cell microarray chip system for accurate, highly sensitive, and rapid diagnosis for malaria in Uganda. Scientific Reports. 2016;**6**(30136):1-9. DOI: 10.1038/srep30136

[13] Lima GFMC et al. Malaria diagnosis from pooled blood samples : Comparative analysis of real-time PCR, nested PCR and immunoassay as a platform for the molecular and

serological diagnosis of malaria on a large-scale. Mem Inst Oswaldo Cruz, Rio Janeiro. 2011;**106**(September): 691-700

[14] Andrade BB et al. Towards a precise test for malaria diagnosis in the Brazilian Amazon: Comparison among field microscopy, a rapid diagnostic test, nested PCR, and a computational expert system based on artificial neural networks. Malaria Journal. 2010;**9**(117): 1-11

[15] Vanessa J et al. Increased frequency of Pfdhps A581G mutation in plasmodium falciparum isolates from Gabonese HIV-infected individuals. Malaria Research Treatment. 2019;**2019** (Article ID 9523259):1-8

[16] Siwal N et al. Malaria diagnosis by PCR revealed the differential distribution of mono and mixed species infections by plasmodium falciparum and *P. vivax* in India. PLoS One. 2018; **13**(3):1-14

[17] Samantaray JC, Ahmed NH. Quantitative Buffy coat analysis effective tool for diagnosing blood parasites. Journal of Clinical Diagnostic Research. 2014;**8**(4):110095. DOI: 10.7860/JCDR/2014/7559.4258

[18] Alias A, Afifi SAB, Zuraidah R, Shukri A, Khairul AA. Malaria diagnosis technique by quantitative Buffy coat. The Medical Journal of Malaysia. 1996; **51**(2):227-231

[19] Singh G, Urhekar AD. Quantitative Buffy coat: A useful tool for diagnosis of malaria. International Journal of Advanced Microbiology and Health Research. 2018;**2**(3):31-36

[20] Kocharekar MM, Sarkar SS, Dasgupta D. Comparative study of modified quantitative Buffy coat and two rapid tests in comparison with peripheral blood smear in malaria diagnosis in Mumbai, India. Journal of Parasitology Research. 2014; **2014**:1-8

[21] Salmani MP, Mindolli PB, Peerapur BV. Comparative study of peripheral blood smear, QBC and antigen detection in malaria diagnosis. Journal of Clinical Diagnostic Research. 2011;**5**(5):967-969

[22] Amir A, Cheong F, De Silva JR, Lau Y. Diagnostic tools in childhood malaria. Parasite Vectors. 2018;**11**(53): 1-12. DOI: 10.1186/s13071-018-2617-y

[23] Waje T. Advances in clinical toxicology malaria tests-DNA PCR and quantitative Buffy coat (QBC). Advances in Clinical Toxicology. 2022;**7**(1):1-5. DOI: 10.23880/act-16000232

[24] Kochareka M, Sarkar S, Dasgupta D, Aigal U. A preliminary comparative report of quantitative buffy coat and modified quantitative buffy coat with peripheral blood smear in malaria diagnosis. Pathogens and Global Health. 2012;**106**(6):335-339. DOI: 10.1179/2047773212Y.0000000024

[25] Sandhya B, S. A. S, Nagaraj ER, Mannur S, Anand S. Laboratory diagnosis of malaria by conventional peripheral blood smear examination with quantitative Buffy coat (QBC) and rapid diagnostic tests (RDT)—A comparative study. International Journal of Collaborative Research on Internal Medicine and Public Health. 2012;**4**(10): 1746-1755

[26] Thiago M-N, Carlos AM, Giorgio Gianini Morbiol EC, Milan LA, Silva DF, Donofrio FC. Improved assessment of accuracy and performance indicators in paper-based ELISA. Analytical Methods.

2017;**9**(18):2613-2758. DOI: 10.1039/c7ay00505a

[27] Doderer C et al. A new ELISA kit which uses a combination of plasmodium falciparum extract and recombinant plasmodium vivax antigens as an alternative to IFAT for detection of malaria antibodies. Malaria Journal. 2007;**6**(19):1-8. DOI: 10.1186/1475-2875-6-19

[28] Akpogheneta OJ et al. Duration of naturally acquired antibody responses to blood-stage plasmodium falciparum is age dependent and antigen-specific. Infection and Immunity. 2008;**76**(4): 1748-1755. DOI: 10.1128/IAI.01333-07

[29] Cao XE, Kim J, Mehta S, Erickson D. Two-color duplex platform for point-of-care Di ff erential detection of malaria and typhoid fever. Analytical Chemistry. 2021;**93**:12175-12180. DOI: 10.1021/acs.analchem.1c03298

[30] Warhurst DC, Williams JE. Laboratory diagnosis of malaria. Journal of Clinical Pathology. 1996;**49**:533-538

[31] Muerhoff AS et al. Detection of Plasmodium falciparum, *P. vivax*, *P. ovale*, and *P. malariae* merozoite surface protein 1-p19 antibodies in human malaria patients and experimentally infected nonhuman primates. Clinical and Vaccine Immunology. 2010;**17**(10): 1631-1638. DOI: 10.1128/CVI.00196-10

[32] Müller-Sienerth N et al. A panel of recombinant proteins from human-infective plasmodium species for serological surveillance. Malaria Journal. 2020;**19**(1):1-15. DOI: 10.1186/s12936-020-3111-5

[33] Thongdee P, Chaijaroenkul W, Kuesap J, Na-Bangchang K. Nested-PCR and a new ELISA-based NovaLisa test kit for malaria diagnosis in an endemic area of Thailand. The Korean Journal of Parasitology. 2014;**52**(4):377-382. DOI: 10.3347/kjp.2014.52.4.377

[34] Duo-quan W, Lin-hua T, Zhen-cheng G, Xiang Z, Man-ni Y. Application of the indirect fluorescent antibody assay in the study of malaria infection in the Yangtze River Three Gorges Reservoir. Malaria Journal. 2009;**7**:1-7. DOI: 10.1186/1475-2875-8-199

[35] Noppadon Tangpukdee SK, Duagdee C, Wilairatana P. Malaria diagnosis: A brief review. The Korean Journal of Parasitology. 2009;**47**(2): 93-102

[36] Boyle MJ et al. IgM in human immunity to plasmodium falciparum malaria. Science Advances. 2019;**5**(9): 1-14. DOI: 10.1126/sciadv.aax4489

[37] Haider F, Ahmad S, Ansari A. Diagnostic performance of the rapid diagnostic test (RDT) and enzyme-linked immunosorbent assay (ELISA) in comparison with microscopy, for malaria. International Journal of Mosquito Research. 2020;**7**(6):33-39

[38] Kitchen AD, Lowe PHJ, Lalloo K, Chiodini PL. Evaluation of a malarial antibody assay for use in the screening of blood and tissue products for clinical use. Vox Sanguinis. 2004;**87**(3): 150-155. DOI: 10.1111/j.1423-0410.2004.00561.x

[39] Van Den Hoogen LL et al. Comparison of commercial ELISA kits to confirm the absence of transmission in malaria elimination settings. Frontiers in Public Health. 2020;**8**(480):1-12. DOI: 10.3389/fpubh.2020.00480

[40] Mangano VD et al. Risk of transfusion-transmitted malaria: Evaluation of commercial ELISA kits for

the detection of anti-plasmodium antibodies in candidate blood donors. Malaria Journal. 2019;**18**(1):1-9. DOI: 10.1186/s12936-019-2650-0

[41] Crowther J. Method in Molecular Biology: The ELISA Guidebook. 2nd ed. Vol. 516. Totuwa, New Jersey: Humana Press; 2009

[42] Johnston SP, Pieniazek NJ, Xayavong MV, Slemenda SB, Wilkins PP, Silva AJ. PCR as a confirmatory technique for laboratory diagnosis of malaria. Journal of Clinical Microbiology. 2006;**44**(3):1087-1089. DOI: 10.1128/JCM.44.3.1087

[43] Sahoo PK, Mohanty DP, Priyadarshini P, Sarangi G. Detection and species determination of malaria parasites by microscopy, antigen detection, polymerase chain reaction, and loop-mediated isothermal amplification assay in a tertiary care hospital. National Journal of Physiology Pharmacy and Pharmacology. 2023;**13** (03):601-606. DOI: 10.5455/njppp.2023.13.01015202319012023

[44] Ascher M et al. Ultrasensitive molecular tests for plasmodium detection: Applicability in control and elimination programs and reference laboratories. Pan American Journal of Public Health. 2022;**46**:1-10. DOI: https://doi.org/10.26633/RPSP.2022.11

[45] Chaudry JZ, Ahmed S, Qureshi TZ, Ali N. Real-time polymerase chain reaction for the detection of malarial parasite. Journal of College of Physicians and Surgeons Pakistan. 2012;**22**(213): 98-100

[46] Parija SC. PCR for diagnosis of malaria. Indian Journal of Medical Research. 2014;**132**:9-10

[47] Smith DM. Using a pooling strategy. American Journal of Tropical Medicine. 2010;**81**(5):754-757. DOI: 10.4269/ajtmh.2009.09-0274.Malaria

[48] Nair CB, Manjula J, Subramani PA. Differential diagnosis of malaria on Truelab Uno 1, a portable, real-time, MicroPCR device for point-of-care applications. PLoS One. 2016;**11**(1):1-14. DOI: 10.1371/journal.pone.0146961

[49] Hayashida K et al. Direct detection of falciparum and non-falciparum malaria DNA from a drop of blood with high sensitivity by the dried- LAMP system. Parasites & Vectors. 2017; **10**(26):1-9. DOI: 10.1186/s13071-016-1949-8

[50] Echeverry DF et al. Human malaria diagnosis using a single-step direct - PCR based on the plasmodium cytochrome oxidase III gene. Malaria Journal. 2016; **15**(128):1-12. DOI: 10.1186/s12936-016-1185-x

[51] Grabias B, Essuman E, Quakyi IA, Kumar S. Sensitive real-time PCR detection of plasmodium falciparum parasites in whole blood by erythrocyte membrane protein 1 gene amplification. Malaria Journal. 2019;**18**(116):1-9. DOI: 10.1186/s12936-019-2743-9

[52] La S, Ponnampalavanar S. Comparison of two nested PCR methods for the detection of human malaria. Tropical Biomedicine. 2013;**30**(3): 459-466

[53] Ugah UI et al. Evaluation of the utility value of three diagnostic methods in the detection of malaria parasites in an endemic area. Malaria Journal. 2017; **16**(189):1-8. DOI: 10.1186/s12936-017-1838-4

[54] Nakatsu M, Kato Y, Komaki-Yasuda K, Perpe J. A novel PCR-based system

for the detection of four species of human malaria parasites and plasmodium knowlesi. PLoS One. 2018; **13**(1):1-15

[55] Snehanshu Shukla HP. Review article. Journal of Evolution of Medical and Dental Sciences. 2013;**2**(28): 5194-5205

[56] WHO. Meeting to Reach Consensus on a Global Dietary Diversity Indicator for Women. 2014. Available from: https://www.fantaproject.org/sites/default/files/resources/WDDP-Meeting-Report-Oct2014.pdf

[57] Hsiang MS, Greenhouse B, Rosenthal PJ. Point of care testing for malaria using LAMP, loop-mediated isothermal amplification. The Journal of Infectious Diseases. 2014;**2014**(210): 1167-1169. DOI: 10.1093/infdis/jiu253

[58] Sattabongkot J, Tsuboi T, Han E, Bantuchai S. Loop-mediated isothermal amplification assay for rapid diagnosis of malaria infections in an area of Endemicity in Thailand. Journal of Clinical Microbiology. 2014;**52**(5): 1471-1477. DOI: 10.1128/JCM.03313-13

[59] Sirichaisinthop J et al. Short report : Evaluation of loop-mediated isothermal amplification (LAMP) for malaria diagnosis in a field setting. The American Journal of Tropical Medicine and Hygiene. 2011;**85**(4):594-596. DOI: 10.4269/ajtmh.2011.10-0676

[60] Ocker R, Chutipongvivate S, Karanis P. Malaria diagnosis by loop-mediated isothermal amplification (LAMP) in. Revista do Instituto de Medicina Tropical. 2016;**58**(271):1-6. DOI: 10.1590/S1678-9946201658027

[61] Tambo M, Id MM, Id DRM. Loop-mediated isothermal amplification (LAMP) and polymerase chain reaction (PCR) as quality assurance tools for rapid diagnostic test (RDT) malaria diagnosis in. PLoS One. 2018;**13**(12):1-8

[62] Lucchi NW et al. Real-time fluorescence loop-mediated isothermal amplification for the diagnosis of malaria. PLoS One. 2010;**5**(10):1-7. DOI: 10.1371/journal.pone.0013733

[63] Akram A. Loop-mediated isothermal amplification (LAMP) for detection of various organisms: A review. Bangladesh Journal of Medical Microbiology. 2017; **11**(2):20-27

[64] Dea-ayuela MA, Galiana-roselló C, Lalatsa A, Serrano DR. Applying loop-mediated isothermal amplification (LAMP) in the Diagno- sis of malaria , Leishmaniasis and Trypanosomiasis as point-of-care tests (POCTs). Current Topics in Medicinal Chemistry. 2018; **18**(10):1-17. DOI: 10.2174/1568026618666181025095735

[65] Wong Y, Othman S, Lau Y, Radu S, Chee H. Loop-mediated isothermal amplification (LAMP): A versatile technique for detection of micro-organisms. Journal of Applied Microbiology. 2017;**124**:626-643. DOI: 10.1111/jam.13647

[66] Zhang J et al. Molecular & Biochemical Parasitology Application of a low-cost, specific, and sensitive loop-mediated isothermal amplification (LAMP) assay to detect plasmodium falciparum imported from Africa. Molecular and Biochemical Parasitology. 2022;**252**(March):111529. DOI: 10.1016/j.molbiopara.2022.111529

[67] Puri M et al. Rapid diagnosis of plasmodium falciparum malaria using an isothermal amplification device. Frontiers in Cellular and Infection Microbiology. 2022;**12**(961832):1-10. DOI: 10.3389/fcimb.2022.961832

[68] Mhlanga N, Cobongela S. Diagnosis of infectious diseases: Tuberculosis, malaria and HIV and aids—A review. Insights in Chemistry and Biochemistry. 2021;**1**(4):1-14. DOI: 10.33552/ICBC.2021.01.000518

[69] Jain P, Chakma B, Patra S, Goswami P. Potential biomarkers and their applications for rapid and reliable detection of malaria. BioMed Research International. 2014;**2014**(Article ID 852645):1-20

[70] Hernández C, Ramírez JD. Air & Water Borne Diseases Molecular Diagnosis of vector-borne parasitic diseases. Air Water Borne Diseases. 2013;**2**(1):1-10. DOI: 10.4172/2167-7719.1000110

[71] Myaing Nyunt J, Pisciotta J, Feldman AB, Thuma P, Scholl PF, Demirev PA, et al. Detection of plasmodium falciparum in pregnancy by laser desorption mass spectrometry. American Journal of Tropical Medicine. 2005;**73**(3):485-490

[72] Sullivan D, Scholl P, Kumar N. Rapid detection of malaria parasites. JOHNS HOPKINS APL Technologu Digest. 2010;**28**(3):232-233

[73] Enyaev YUAM et al. Preclinical photoacoustic models: Application for ultrasensitive single cell malaria diagnosis in large vein and artery. Biomedical Optics Express. 2016;**7**(9):1458-1462

[74] Negi A, Mirdha BR, Arulselvi S, Singh A, Patel SS. Evaluation of an automated, high throughput Flowcytometry based technique for diagnosis of malaria. International Journal of Current Microbiology and Applied Science. 2018;**7**(06):941-951

[75] Roobsoong W et al. A rapid sensitive, flow cytometry-based method for the detection of plasmodium vivax -infected blood cells. Malaria Journal. 2014;**13**(55):1-11

[76] Harba NM, Rady AA, Khalefa KA. RESEARCH ARTICLE PUJ evaluation of flow cytometry as a diagnostic method for detection of Giardia lamblia in comparison to IFAT and other conventional staining techniques in Fecal samples. PUJ. 2012;**5**(2):165-174

[77] Henel G, Schmitz JL. Basic theory and clinical applications of flow cytometry. Labmedicine. 2007;**38**(7):428-436. DOI: 10.1309/GHLEWLV0CD8025JL

[78] Chaturvedi A, Gorthi SS. Automated blood sample preparation unit (ABSPU) for portable microfluidic flow cytometry. Slas-Technology. 2017;**22**(1):73-80. DOI: 10.1177/2211068216663604

[79] Aninagyei E, Abraham J, Atiiga P, Antwi SD, Bamfo S, Acheampong DO. Evaluating the potential of using urine and saliva specimens for malaria diagnosis in suspected patients in Ghana. Malaria Journal. 2020;**19**(349):1-9. DOI: 10.1186/s12936-020-03427-x

[80] Oguonu T, Shu E. The performance evaluation of a urine malaria test (UMT) kit for the diagnosis of malaria in individuals with fever in south-East Nigeria: A cross-sectional analytical study. Malaria Journal. 2014;**12**(403):1-6. DOI: 10.1186/1475-2875-13-403

[81] Nwakanma DC et al. Quantitative detection of plasmodium falciparum DNA in saliva, blood, and urine. The Journal of Infectious Diseases. 2009;**199**:1567-1574. DOI: 10.1086/598856

[82] Anchinmane VT, Shedge RT. Detection of malarial parasite in the

urine of malaria patients: A future diagnostic approach. International Journal of Research Medicine and Science. 2016;**4**(5):1702-1705

[83] Danwang C, Noubiap JJ, Souopgui J, Gaudart J, Yombi JC, Robert A. Accuracy of malaria diagnostic tests invasively collected performed on non-samples: A systematic review and meta-analysis. BMJ Global Health. 2021;**6**(e005634): 1-7. DOI: 10.1136/bmjgh-2021-005634

[84] Shah A, Shethwala ND, Shah TA. Urine analysis findings of malaria patients attending tertiary care hospital of North Gujarat. International Journal of Medicine and Research. 2016;**5**(4):2-5

[85] Tobón-castaño A, Escobar SB, Castro CG. Urinalysis and clinical correlations in patients with *P. vivax* or *P. falciparum* malaria from Colombia. Hindawi Journal of Tropical Medicine. 2017;**2017**(7868535):1-12. DOI: 10.1155/2017/7868535

[86] Tao D et al. A saliva-based rapid test to quantify the infectious subclinical malaria parasite reservoir. Science Transitional Medicine. 2019;**11** (eaan4479):1-13

[87] Siddig H, Saber S, El-ashy M. Original article urine-based rapid diagnostic test for diagnosis of plasmodium falciparum malaria. Microbes Infectious Diseases. 2023;**4**(1): 268-275. DOI: 10.21608/MID.2022.150231.1347

[88] Gopal A, Kumari P, Kumar A, Satpathi S, Kumar A. The sensitivity and specificity of a urine-based rapid diagnostic test for the diagnosis of plasmodium falciparum in a malaria endemic area in Odisha, India. Pathogens and Global Health. 2017; **111**(7):1-5. DOI: 10.1080/20477724.2017.1380945

[89] Pradhan N, Hazra RK. Can a non-invasive urine-based test become the next-generation diagnostic tool for malaria? Le Infez. Med. 2018;**3**:199-203

[90] Putaporntip C, Buppan P, Jongwutiwes S. Improved performance with saliva and urine as alternative DNA sources for malaria diagnosis by mitochondrial DNA-based PCR assays. Clinical Microbiology and Infection. 2011;**17**:1484-1491

[91] Abiodun A, Olugbenga A, Kazeem A, Olusola GG. Detection of malaria parasite protein in urine of patients with acute uncomplicated malaria using rapid diagnostic test kits. Journal of Microbiology and Infectious Disease. 2022;**12**(August):97-107. DOI: 10.5799/jmid.1176524

[92] Chai HC, Chai KH. Urine and saliva : Relevant specimens for malaria diagnosis ? Diagnostics. 2022;**12**(2989): 1-18

[93] Costa GL, Anete D, Alvarenga M. Improving the molecular diagnosis of malaria : Droplet digital PCR-based method using saliva as a DNA source. Frontiers in Genetics. 2022;**13**(May): 1-12. DOI: 10.3389/fmicb.2022.882530

Section 4

Malaria Treatment

Chapter 7

Malaria Treatment Landscape: Current Trends and Future Directions

Eulambius Mathias Mlugu

Abstract

Malaria control relies partly on effective case treatment, with Artemisinin-based combination therapy (ACT) being a cornerstone strategy. ACTs have revolutionized malaria treatment by offering remarkable efficacy and bolstering disease control efforts. They demonstrate exceptional effectiveness against both falciparum and non-falciparum malaria, rendering them suitable for all malaria variants. However, a declining malaria transmission rate introduces a new concern, a heightened risk of severe malaria among the elderly due to fading premunition. An important advancement in malaria management is the deployment of artesunate for severe cases. Given the decreasing transmission rates, a comprehensive control package encompassing disease control and elimination is essential. Primaquine has proven to be effective in curtailing malaria transmission, positioning it as a key component in elimination strategies. In pursuit of malaria eradication, optimization of integrated tools for mass drug administration and chemoprevention initiatives targeting vulnerable populations is crucial. As the development of new antimalarial drugs remains uncertain, securing the longevity of ACTs necessitates innovative approaches and substantial investments. Looking forward, addressing pivotal challenges such as drug resistance, sub-optimal plasma drug exposure, diagnostic insensitivity, and sub-standard medications is paramount. By tackling these challenges head-on, the global community can bolster malaria control and work toward its eventual eradication.

Keywords: malaria, rapid diagnostic tests, ACTs, resistance, chemoprevention

1. Introduction

Malaria remains a significant global health concern, particularly in the tropical and subtropical regions of Africa. Six species of Plasmodium parasites are known to cause malaria in humans transmitted through the bites of infected Anopheles mosquitoes [1]. *Plasmodium falciparum* is the predominant causative agent of the disease in Africa and the most virulent species. Other species are less virulent and commonly found in Southeast Asia and Western Pacific. The global burden of malaria has substantially declined as compared to the levels at the beginning of the new millennium in the year 2000 [2]. The malaria control achievements were contributed by financial investments and innovative approaches fueled by the Millennium Development

IntechOpen

Goals and later Sustainable Development Goals (SDGs) [3, 4]. Despite the substantial decline, hundreds of millions of people are still affected by malaria each year, leading to hundreds of thousands of deaths globally [5].

Malaria treatment is a vital component among the efforts for the control and elimination of the disease. Effective treatment is crucial not only for reducing morbidity and mortality but also for controlling the spread of the disease. The treatment of malaria involves a multi-faceted approach, including the use of antimalarial medications, supportive care, and preventive strategies. The cornerstone of malaria management is the use of antimalarial drugs, which directly target the Plasmodium parasite. The choice of antimalarial drugs depends on various factors, including the severity of the infection, the type of Plasmodium species, the patient's age, the likely pattern of susceptibility to antimalarial drugs, the cost, availability of such drugs, and geographical location. For this reason, recommendations vary according to geographic region and are usually under constant review.

Artemisinin which forms the current mainstay of antimalarial treatment is derived from the leaves of a Chinese herb known as *Artemisia annua* [6]. Its derivatives include dihydroartemisinin, artesunate, and artemether. Artemisinin-based combination therapies (ACTs) are the first-line treatment for uncomplicated falciparum malaria [7]. ACTs combine an artemisinin derivative, which rapidly reduces the parasite load, with a long-acting partner drug that clears the remaining parasites from the bloodstream. The long-acting partner drugs belong to synthetic 4-aminoquinoline (amodiaquine and piperaquine), aryl amino alcohol (mefloquine, lumefantrine, and halofantrine), and aminoacridine (pyronaridine). The combination of these drugs helps to prevent the development of drug resistance and ensures a higher cure rate. ACTs or chloroquine are equally effective in the treatment of infections caused by non-falciparum species [7]. *Plasmodium vivax and Plasmodium ovale* can form dormant liver-stage parasites referred to as hypnozoites [8]. To prevent relapses due to hypnozoites, additional drugs like primaquine or tafenoquine are used to target these latent forms after ACT or chloroquine [9].

Chemoprevention has emerged as a promising strategy to complement existing global malaria control strategies and proved to be effective, especially in vulnerable populations. In Africa, where *P. falciparum* is still sensitive, dihydroartemisinin-piperaquine (DHP) is explored for use in chemoprevention approaches targeting the elimination of malaria, though caution needs to be taken to prevent resistance development. However, resistance to DHP is widespread in the Great Mekong region, Southeast Asia [10]. Innovative researches are needed to generate further evidence on the optimal regimes, especially among the existing tools for effective chemoprevention.

Effective malaria treatment relies on early diagnosis and the use of appropriate antimalarial drugs. Prompt and accurate diagnosis ensures timely administration of drugs, reduces the severity of the disease, and prevents complications and deaths. In endemic regions, rapid diagnostic tests (RDTs) have revolutionized malaria diagnosis by providing quick and reliable results without the need for sophisticated laboratory equipment. Nevertheless, lower sensitivities [11] and deletion of *P. falciparum* histidine- rich protein 2 and 3, the target proteins in RDTs [12] challenge the effective diagnosis and treatment of malaria. Other challenges like drug resistance, limited healthcare access, co-infections, and socioeconomic factors pose significant obstacles in combatting malaria effectively [13]. Strengthening malaria treatment efforts will make significant strides toward eliminating the global burden of this devastating disease. This chapter provides a comprehensive insight into the current approaches for the management of malaria focusing on key therapeutics and chemoprophylaxis options, as well as challenges and future direction for strengthening the treatment and control strategies toward malaria eradication.

2. Malaria treatment approaches

Before 2006, malaria treatment regimens consisted of monotherapies. During that time, chloroquine and amodiaquine were widely used against infections caused by all types of parasite species. In some endemic areas, chloroquine is now less effective due to widespread resistance [14]. However, it is still utilized in other areas where the Plasmodium species are susceptible to their action, especially against the non-*falciparum* species. Amodiaquine is still available as a partner drug in combination therapy. The antifolate sulfadoxine-pyrimethamine (SP) was an effective and well-tolerated antimalarial drug given as a single dose. SP is also a partner drug in combination therapy although the widely spread resistance limits its use for malaria treatment in some areas. However, it is recommended for malaria intermittent preventive treatment (IPT) in endemic areas [15].

Following the WHO's first edition of the Guidelines for malaria treatment in 2006 [16], many countries changed the malaria treatment regimen from monotherapy to combination therapy. ACTs are highly effective in treating uncomplicated malaria caused by *Plasmodium falciparum* [17] and non-falciparum malaria infections [18]. The combination offers several advantages over monotherapies. ACTs achieve faster parasite clearance and reduce the risk of treatment failure compared to monotherapy. Combining artemisinin derivatives with a partner drug that has a different mechanism of action, help to delay the development of drug resistance. The combination of artemisinin with another antimalarial drug often enhances the overall therapeutic effect thus providing a synergistic effect. The partner drug may have a longer half-life, ensuring continuous parasite clearance and reducing the chances of recrudescence [19]. By rapidly reducing the number of parasites in the blood, ACTs contribute to reduce the transmission and prevalence of malaria in communities.

2.1 Types of ACTs

The World Health Organization (WHO) recommends six ACTs for the treatment of uncomplicated falciparum malaria [7] namely:

A. Artemether-lumefantrine

B. Artesunate-mefloquine

C. Artesunate-amodiaquine

D. Artesunate-sulfadoxine-pyrimethamine

E. Dihydroartemisinin-piperaquine

F. Artesunate-pyronaridine

2.2 Mechanism of action for antimalarial drugs

Artemisinin and its derivatives exhibit potent antimalarial activity by targeting the Plasmodium parasites during their asexual blood stage. The mode of action involves the production of reactive oxygen species, which damage the parasite's cellular components, leading to its death [20]. Artemisinin derivatives have a rapid onset of action, reducing the parasite load quickly.

The partner drugs in ACTs have a longer half-life and eliminate the remaining parasites. They target blood stage parasites although the exact mechanism is unknown. The current knowledge suggests that lumefantrine acts by forming a complex with hemin and inhibits β-hematin formation and consequently inhibits nucleic acid and protein synthesis. Aminoquinoline, aminoacridine, and bisquinoline partner drugs are hypothesized to have a similar mechanism through binding to heme and arrest the polymerization of a toxic haematin resulting in its accumulation in the erythrocytes destroying the parasites [21]. The antifolates antimalarial drugs work through the inhibition of key enzymes involved in the folate pathways. Sulfadoxine inhibits dihydropteroate synthase (DHPS), an important enzyme in folate synthesis by the parasites [22]. On the flip side, pyrimethamine competitively inhibits a key enzyme for the production of tetrahydrofolate, dihydrofolate reductase (DHFR) which is a crucial co-factor needed by the parasites for the biosynthesis of nucleotides and proteins [23].

2.3 Treatment regimens for uncomplicated malaria

Artemether-lumefantrine (ALu) is the first-line treatment policy in most African countries. It is the most commonly used ACT available in a fixed-dose combination. Each tablet contains 20 mg of artemether and 120 mg of Lumefantrine. The recommended dose is 1.4–4 mg/kg for artemether and 10–16 mg/kg for lumefantrine. However, it is conveniently administered in a pre-defined weight band. Patients weighing 5–14 kg receive one tablet (20 mg artemether/120 mg Lumefantrine), 15–24 kg receive two tablets, 25–34 kg receive three tablets, and > 34 kg receive four tablets given twice daily for three consecutive days [24]. One tablet formulation containing 80 mg of artemether and 480 mg of lumefantrine is also available for patients weighing >34 kg to reduce pill burden. Formulations for pediatric patients are also available in the form of dispersible tablets [25]. The first dose is usually administered at the health facility as a direct observed therapy (DOT). Recent evidence indicates that ALu is safe in pregnancy and is recommended in all trimesters [26] making one regimen for the general population, children, and pregnant women.

DHP is also one of the first-line treatment policies in some African countries. It is very well-tolerated and available in a fixed dose combination containing 40 mg dihydroartemisinin and 320 mg piperaquine per tablet. Pediatric formulations are available in a strength of 20 mg dihydroartemisinin and 160 mg piperaquine per tablet. The dose regimen for children weighing <25 kg is 4 mg of dihydroartemisinin per kg body weight and 24 mg of piperaquine per kg body weight given once daily for three consecutive days. For children weighing ≥25 kg and adults, the dose is 4 mg of dihydroartemisinin per kg body weight and 18 mg of piperaquine per kg body weight given once daily for three consecutive days [27]. However, in resource-limited countries, weight-based dosing is a challenge, thus adults receive a three-day course of three tablets daily. Resistance to DHP is widely spread in the Great Mekong region and necessitated the removal of this regimen as the first-line policy [10].

In Southeast Asia, the first-line policy is artesunate-amodiaquine (AS-AQ) which is also the first-line policy in some West African countries. AS-AQ is available in a fixed dose formulation containing different strengths of 25/67.5, 50/135, and 100/270 mg of artesunate/amodiaquine, respectively [28]. Artesunate 50 mg and amodiaquine 135 mg are also available as separate formulations. AS-AQ is given once daily for three consecutive days at a dose of 4 mg/kg for artesunate and 10 mg/kg of amodiaquine. For convenient dosing, AS-AQ is also given in weight bands where, children weighing between 4.5 to <9 kg receive one tablet (25/67.5 mg) once daily for 3 days, 9 to <18 kg receive one tablet (50/135 mg), 18 to <36 kg receive one tablet (100/270 mg) once daily for 3 days and those weighing ≥36 kg and adults receive two tablets (100/270 mg) once daily for 3 days [28].

Artesunate mefloquine is available in a separate formulation. One formulation contains 50 mg of artesunate and the other 250 mg of mefloquine base. The recommended dose is 4 mg/kg/day for artesunate given once daily for 3 days and 25 mg/kg of mefloquine divided over 2 days as 15 mg/kg and 10 mg/kg given on the second and third days [29]. Artesunate-SP is available on a separate tablet. However, due to widespread resistance to SP, this regimen is not used in some countries. Artesunate-pyronaridine is a recently introduced ACT regimen available in a fixed dose formulation containing 60 mg of artesunate and 180 mg of pyronaridine as a salt. The fixed-dose formulation is indicated for children with 20 kg body weight and above. Patients weighing 20 to <24 kg receive one tablet, 24 to <45 kg receive two tablets, 45 to <65 kg receive three tablets, and ≥ 65 kg receive four tablets once daily for 3 days. For children with <20 kg body weight, the granular pediatric formulation is available in a sachet packaging containing 20 mg of artesunate and 60 mg of pyronaridine tetraphosphate [30]. Children weighing 5 to <8 kg receive one sachet, 8 to <15 kg receive two sachets, and 15 to <29 kg receive three sachets. Nevertheless, the deployment of Artesunate-pyronaridine has not been expanded in many countries. It is essential to follow the prescribed dosage and complete the full course of treatment to ensure effectiveness and reduce the risk of developing drug resistance.

Chloroquine is recommended for the treatment of blood stage uncomplicated infection with a non-falciparum parasite. Chloroquine is formulated in tablet form with a strength of 250 mg per tablet. The prescribed dosage regimen for adults involves an initial dose of four tablets (250 mg per tablet), followed by two tablets after 6 hours, followed by a maintenance dose of two tablets daily for 2 days [31]. For pediatric patients, the recommended chloroquine dosage involves an initial dose of 10 mg base/kg then, a follow-up dose of 5 mg base/kg after 6 hours, followed by a maintenance dose of 5 mg base/kg once daily for 2 days. Children aged 1–4 years receive an initial dose of one tablet, followed by half a tablet after 6 hours, and then half a tablet once daily for 2 days. Children aged 5–8 years receive two tablets for the initial dose, followed by one tablet after 6 hours, and then one tablet once daily for 2 days. Children aged 9–14 years should take three tablets initially, followed by one and a half tablets after 6 hours, and then one and a half tablets once daily for 2 days [31].

ACTs have demonstrated good efficacy and safety for non-falciparum infections [18] and are used for the treatment of the same making one therapeutic approach for all Plasmodium infections. Infections with *P. vivax* and *P. ovale* exist as hypnozoites that survive in the liver and may result in relapse. Since most antimalarial drugs act on the blood stage of the parasite, primaquine given at a dose of 0.25 mg/kg daily for seven or 14 days is recommended to eliminate hypnozoites in the liver after a full course of chloroquine or ACT [32]. The risk of recrudescence is lower with DHP than ALu and decreases with additional primaquine [33]. Recently, tefenoquine a long-acting and well-tolerated member of 8-aminoquinoline given as a single dose proved to be an alternative to primaquine as it outweighs adherence problems [34]. A low dose of primaquine is also effective against the transmissibility of falciparum mature gametocytes interrupting malaria transmission, especially in areas of low transmission intensities requiring elimination [35]. A single dose of 0.25 mg/kg primaquine for falciparum infections after a three-day course of ACT reduces gametocytemia thus blocking the transmission of the disease [35]. Primaquine is known to cause hemolysis in individuals with glucose-6-phosphate dehydrogenase (G6PD) deficiency, making testing for G6PD deficiency important before administering the drug. In resource-constrained countries, G6PD testing is not feasible in routine settings. However, recent evidence indicates that a single dose of primaquine as recommended by the WHO is safe even among G6PD-deficit patients with minimal reduction in Hemoglobin [36, 37]. The availability of simple and cost-effective G6PD tests for routine use in the future will aid in the safe management of malaria.

2.4 Treatment regimens and management of severe malaria

Severe malaria is a life-threatening medical emergency caused primarily by the *P. falciparum* parasite. It is a significant public health concern, particularly in regions with high malaria transmission rates. With the decreasing burden of malaria, cases of severe malaria are also rare although, may be problematic in the older population as primunition wanes. Prompt and appropriate treatment is essential to reduce mortality and morbidity associated with severe malaria. Management of severe malaria aims immediately to reduce the parasite load, manage the symptoms, manage the associated complications, and proper supportive care.

Artesunate, a water-soluble drug can rapidly reduce parasite load and improve survival rates in patients with severe malaria and is the first-line treatment for severe malaria [7]. It can be administered intravenously or intramuscularly for critically ill patients and is available in both parenteral and rectal formulations for use in resource-limited settings. Following initial treatment with intravenous or intramuscular artesunate, a full course of ACT is given to clear any remaining parasites and to complete the treatment. ACTs, such as ALu or AS-AQ, are highly effective and help to prevent the development of drug resistance. The choice of ACT may depend on local drug resistance patterns and individual patient factors.

In addition to antimalarial medications, supportive care plays a critical role in the management of severe malaria. Severe malaria often presents with complications including anemia, metabolic acidosis, and multi-organ dysfunction, which require specific interventions. Intravenous fluids and electrolyte management are essential to maintain hydration and correct any imbalances. Malaria-associated mortalities occur with admission of <3 g/dL of hemoglobin thus immediate blood transfusions may be necessary [37]. In resource-limited countries, health facilities in rural settings are not sufficient to provide blood transfusion services in addition to poor infrastructure for a quick referral system. This contributes to malaria-associated severe anemia causing mortalities, especially in children. Monitoring of vital signs, such as blood pressure, heart rate, and oxygen saturation, is vital to detect any deterioration promptly. Fever, discomfort, and pain are common symptoms of severe malaria requiring the use of antipyretics, such as paracetamol. Additionally, appropriate analgesics may be needed to manage pain and reduce distress in patients. Frequent monitoring of patients with severe malaria is crucial to assess treatment response and detect any potential complications. Parasitemia usually remains high for about 48 hours thus serial blood smears should be examined to evaluate the reduction in parasite density. Laboratory investigations, including complete blood count, liver and renal function tests, and coagulation profiles, should be performed regularly to identify and manage any adverse effects or complications. Cerebral malaria leading to seizures is a common complication of severe malaria, particularly in young children thus anticonvulsants, such as diazepam or phenobarbital are administered [38]. However, caution should be exercised with the use of diazepam to prevent respiratory depression, especially in critically ill patients. Severe malaria can lead to hypoglycemia, especially in children thus monitoring of blood glucose is also important. Intravenous glucose supplementation may be needed in managing and preventing life-threatening low blood sugar levels.

2.5 Efficacy of antimalarials and drug resistance

To inform policy decisions, WHO recommends regular monitoring of antimalarial drugs through therapeutic efficacy studies (TES). The outcomes of TES, include clinical and parasitological responses monitored for a minimum of 28 days for drugs with elimination half-lives of less than 7 days (lumefantrine, amodiaquine, and artemisinin derivatives). For antimalarial drugs with longer elimination half-lives such as piperaquine and mefloquine longer periods of at least 42 days are recommended [39]. Responses can be regarded as adequate clinical and parasitological responses characterized by the absence of parasitemia on day 28 (day 42) irrespective of axillary temperature. It can be also regarded as early treatment failure (ETF) defined by higher parasitemia on days 1, 2, and 3 as compared to the levels on day 0 with an axillary temperature of ≥37.5°C or late clinical failure (LCF) characterized by danger signs, presence of parasitemia between day 4 and day 28 (42) with the axillary temperature of ≥37.5°C. Additionally, late parasitological failure is characterized by the presence of parasitemia on any day between day 7 and day 28 (day 42). An efficacy rate of at least 90% for ACTs is deemed sufficiently acceptable in therapeutics [39].

Several TES from areas where resistance to ACTs has not been reported have consistently reported acceptable efficacy (≥90%). ALu is particularly effective in regions where *P. falciparum* is still sensitive and demonstrated an overall cure rate of about 98% in endemic regions [19]. In sub-Saharan Africa, few studies have reported ≥10% therapeutic failure for ALu in some countries [19]. Equally, AS-AQ has a high cure rate with an overall efficacy of 98.4% for uncomplicated malaria, making it an important tool in the fight against malaria in regions where drug-resistant strains are a concern. Similar to ALu and AS-AQ, DHP has a high cure rate with an overall efficacy of 99.4% for uncomplicated malaria [40]. It is well-tolerated by most patients and has been widely used in areas where malaria is endemic. It is important to note that the efficacy of antimalarial drugs can vary depending on the geographical location due to the development of drug-resistant strains of the malaria parasite. Therefore, it's essential to monitor drug efficacy regularly and update treatment guidelines accordingly.

The efficacy of controlling malaria is jeopardized by the presence of antimalarial resistance. Therapeutic Efficacy Studies (TES) constitute one approach to track the development of resistance to antimalarial drugs. Elevated instances of treatment ineffectiveness resulting from diminished drug responsiveness might be linked to the emergence of resistance. Additional conventional methods encompass the surveillance of genetic markers linked to drug resistance. Mutation in *PfKelch13* gene is associated with reduced parasite clearance and is used to monitor artemisinin resistance [41]. On the other hand, mutations occurring in the *Pfcrt* transporter, as well as in the *Pfmdr* gene, have led to the development of resistance against chloroquine and its structurally related antimalarials [42]. In the *Pfcrt* gene, mutations are prominent within positions 72–76 among most *P. falciparum strains* causing resistance to 4-aminoquinolines. An increase in *Pfplasmepsin* 2/3 copy numbers as well as mutations occurring in the *Pfcrt* transporter are associated with piperaquine resistance [42, 43]. Resistance to mefloquine and lumefantrine is largely associated with an increase in the copy number of the wild-type *Pfmdr* gene [43]. Meanwhile, resistance to atovaquone emerges readily due to mutations occurring in the mitochondrial multicopy cytochrome b gene specifically at position 268, commonly Y268S or Y268N [43]. The prevalence of *PfKelch13* mutation associated with partial artemisinin resistance is high in Southeast Asia, particularly in the Great Mekong sub-regions of Myanmar and Cambodia, and is spreading to Papua New Guinea [44]. The widespread resistance to DHP led to change in the first-line treatment policy in this region [10]. In the African region, *PfKelch13* mutations have emerged in Uganda, Eritrea and Rwanda [13]. Parasite resistance to antimalarial drugs is associated with reduced parasite clearance.

Mutations within the *dhfr* gene (S108N, N51I, C59R) that encodes the drug target dihydrofolate reductase, result in resistance to pyrimethamine in both *P. falciparum* and *P. vivax*, rendering the drug less effective against these parasites [45]. Similarly, the resistance of both *P. falciparum* and *P. vivax* to sulfadoxine is attributed to mutations accumulating in the *dhps* gene, which is responsible for encoding the drug target dihydropteroate synthase. Notable mutations within this gene include A437G, K540E, and A581G [45]. The combination of these mutations compromises the efficacy of SP. In the WHO eastern Mediterranean region, the widespread resistance to SP necessitated the change of policy to ALu from AS + SP. In addition, the widespread parasite resistance to SP in sub-Saharan Africa impedes the efficiency of SP to clear parasitemia and prevent new infections [46].

2.6 Safety profile of ACTs

Artemisinin derivatives, including artemether, dihydroartemisinin, and artesunate, have demonstrated a favorable safety profile. The most commonly reported adverse events are mild and self-limiting, including nausea, vomiting, dizziness, and headaches. These side effects are generally well-tolerated and rarely lead to treatment discontinuation [47]. However, some patients may experience more severe adverse reactions, such as allergic reactions or anaphylaxis, though these instances are exceedingly rare.

The safety profile of partner drugs in ACTs varies depending on the specific drug used. Lumefantrine, amodiaquine and piperaquine are among the most commonly used partner drugs. Lumefantrine is generally well-tolerated, with gastrointestinal disturbances (e.g., diarrhea) being the most commonly reported adverse events [48]. Concerns have been raised about cardiac safety, particularly in patients with pre-existing cardiac conditions or prolonged QT intervals, but these events are rare and often not directly attributed to lumefantrine [49]. Amodiaquine has a well-documented safety profile and is generally considered safe for use. However, it may cause adverse effects such as hepatotoxicity, which can be severe but is rare. Amodiaquine is known to cause hemolysis in individuals with G6PD deficiency. Piperaquine is well-tolerated, and its safety profile is generally favorable. However, there have been isolated reports of rare adverse events, including cardiovascular events and QT interval prolongation, especially when used at high doses [50].

The safety of ACTs in pregnant women and young children is of paramount importance. Studies have shown that ACTs are safe and effective during pregnancy when used as recommended [26]. Pregnant women with malaria are at an increased risk of drug-related adverse outcomes, but the benefits of treating malaria with ACTs outweigh the potential risks. Similarly, ACTs are equally safe and effective in treating malaria in children, contributing to the reduction of malaria-related mortality in this vulnerable population [51].

3. Chemoprevention of malaria

Chemoprevention involves the administration of a full course of antimalarial drugs to vulnerable populations as a preventive measure. The rationale behind chemoprevention lies in its ability to proactively target malaria parasites during their lifecycle, thereby preventing infection, reducing parasite reservoirs, and subsequently decreasing the risk of transmission. This approach is particularly valuable for high-risk populations, including pregnant women, young children, and travelers visiting malaria-endemic regions. Chemoprevention of malaria has demonstrated its potential as a complementary strategy to conventional malaria control measures. By effectively targeting high-risk populations and interrupting parasite transmission, chemoprevention holds the promise of reducing malaria-related morbidity and mortality.

Pregnant women, in particular, are at increased risk of malaria and adverse pregnancy outcomes due to pregnant-associated immune modulation and the preferential of falciparum parasites to the placenta [52]. Most of the infected women at their first antenatal care clinic have asymptomatic parasitemia [53]. Chemoprevention is therefore a vital intervention to protect both maternal and fetal health. Intermittent Preventive Treatment in Pregnancy (IPTp) involves the administration of a full treatment course of an antimalarial drug during antenatal care visits, irrespective of whether the pregnant woman shows symptoms or has a confirmed infection. SP has been the mainstay for IPTp due to its safety profile and effectiveness against the adverse effects of malaria in pregnancy [54]. The efficiency of SP in the prevention of parasitemia and placental malaria is compromised due to widespread parasite resistance to the drug [46]. However, taking at least three doses of SP during pregnancy is associated with improved birth weight [55] which is explained by the non-malaria effects of SP [56]. IPTp with DHP has recently shown superior efficacy against parasitemia and placental malaria than SP [57]. Future studies need to explore the efficacy and safety of combined DHP and SP for IPTp. IPT with SP has also been recommended to children considering the feasibility of providing it with a routine expanded program for immunization. In addition, Seasonal Malaria Chemoprevention (SMC) using AQ with SP is effectively implemented in endemic areas with high seasonal malaria transmission [58]. In eastern Africa where SP resistance is widespread, SMC with DHP is explored [58, 59].

Mass Drug Administration (MDA) involves administering antimalarial drugs to entire populations in high-transmission settings, regardless of individual infection status. This approach aims to reduce the overall parasite burden in the community and consequently, interrupt transmission. While MDA has shown promising results, its implementation requires careful consideration of factors such as drug resistance and feasibility. With the longest half-life of piperaquine which provides extended prophylaxis, DHP is an ideal option for elimination strategies including MDA [60]. In target areas for elimination, MDA with ACTs demonstrated lower incidences and prevalence of parasitemia [61]. Travelers to malaria-endemic regions can take prophylactic antimalarial medications to prevent infection. Several antimalarial medications, such as mefloquine, atovaquone-proguanil, doxycycline, and primaquine, may be prescribed depending on the specific circumstances, including the region of travel and drug resistance patterns.

While a chemopreventive drug regimen is crucial for malaria control and elimination strategies, consistent adherence to the drug is the main challenge for its effectiveness. Non-adherence can reduce the protective effect and contribute to the emergence of drug resistance. The future of malaria chemoprevention control is promising. Ongoing research should focus on optimizing existing strategies and exploring new drug combinations and delivery methods. Additionally, advancements in molecular diagnostics and genetic surveillance will enable real-time monitoring of drug resistance, allowing for timely adjustments to treatment regimens. Furthermore, targeted chemoprevention based on individual risk profiles may become a reality as we gain a better understanding of the host-parasite interactions that drive severe disease outcomes.

4. Disposition of antimalarial drugs

Understanding the pharmacokinetics of antimalarial drugs is crucial for optimizing treatment regimens, ensuring therapeutic efficacy, successful outcomes in malaria management, and preventing drug resistance. The disposition of antimalarial drugs is a complex process that significantly influences their therapeutic effectiveness and the development of drug resistance. In addition, consideration of individual patient factors and potential drug interactions is essential for tailoring antimalarial therapy and reducing the global burden of malaria effectively. Most commonly, antimalarial drugs are administered orally, and their bioavailability is influenced by factors such as food intake and the presence of drug transporters in the gastrointestinal tract [61, 62]. ACTs taken with fatty meal especially milk has been shown to improve their systemic exposure [63]. The extensive distribution of some antimalarial, like chloroquine, contributes to their ability to target malaria parasites in various tissues. The knowledge of antimalarial drug disposition allows the design of appropriate dosing regimens.

The liver primarily carries out the metabolism of many antimalarial drugs through various enzymatic pathways, including cytochrome P450 enzymes. Artemisinin, artesunate, and artemether are metabolized by various CYP enzymes to a potent active metabolite dihydroartemisinin (**Figure 1**). These enzymes are polymorphic and genetic variations in these enzymes can lead to inter-individual differences in drug metabolism, influencing drug efficacy and toxicity [64]. The role of genetic variations in *CYP3A4* the main metabolic pathway for most antimalarial drugs on their dispositions has not been documented. Genetic variation in *CYP3A5* is associated with lower lumefantrine plasma concentrations and treatment failure [65]. Sub-optimal drug concentrations due to poor adherence or altered pharmacokinetics may provide selective pressure for the emergence of drug-resistant malaria parasites. Continued research in this field will contribute to the development of more effective and targeted antimalarial treatment strategies.

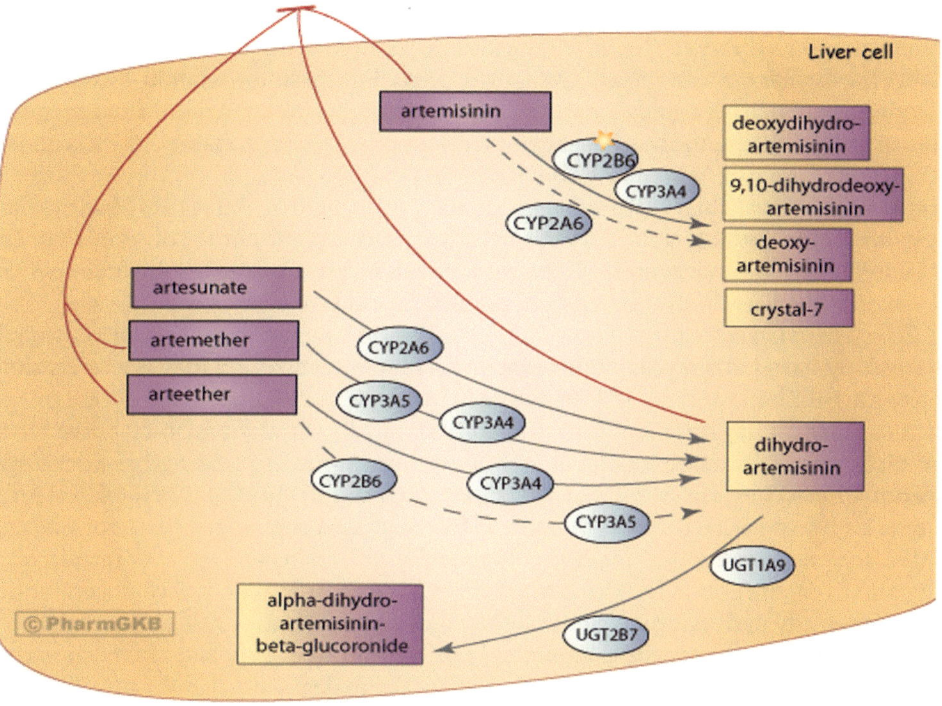

Figure 1.
Metabolic pathways for artemisinin derivatives. Source: https://www.pharmgkb.org/pathway/PA165378192.

5. Challenges and future perspective in the management of malaria

Although progress has been made in malaria control efforts over the years, numerous challenges persist, hindering the effective treatment and management of the disease. One of the most critical challenges in malaria treatment is the emergence and spread of drug-resistant strains of the malaria parasite, particularly *P. falciparum*, which is responsible for the majority of malaria-related deaths. Resistance to antimalarial drugs like chloroquine and SP has been documented in many regions worldwide, limiting treatment options and compromising treatment efficacy. Resistance to artemisinin forming the current treatment regimen has also surfaced in Southeast Asia [66]. Delayed parasite clearance and treatment failures have been observed in some regions. The emergency of artemisinin resistance has been reported in some African countries [13]. The threat of further drug resistance underscores the urgency of developing and deploying new antimalarial drugs. Regular monitoring of drug resistance is essential for maintaining treatment efficacy. Several approaches for mitigating antimalarial resistance are warranted. The availability of different types of ACTs provides an opportunity for further research aiming to mitigate resistance development. Future studies should generate evidence on the effectiveness of multiple first-line drugs and the use of triple artemisinin combination treatments, (TACTs) which combine artemisinin derivatives with two slowly eliminated antimalarial drugs for mitigating drug resistance [67].

Sub-optimal antimalarial plasma exposure resulting in treatment failure is another challenge facing the effective treatment of malaria. Sub-optimal drug concentrations occur in pregnant women possibly due to pregnancy-related increased CYP enzyme activity [68]. Children also have higher clearance of antimalarial drugs leading to sub-therapeutic concentrations [69, 70]. The existence of high-efficacy ACTs provides a chance for further optimization of dosage regimens. Future studies should evaluate the effectiveness of increasing doses or dosing durations, especially in children and pregnant women. Furthermore, the burden of sub-standard drugs in sub-Saharan Africa is under-estimated but contributes to sub-optimal plasma drug exposure and compromises the treatment of malaria. In sub-Saharan Africa, it is estimated that about 19% of antimalarial drugs are falsified or sub-standard with an estimated economic burden of more than US 10 billion [71]. The weak control of pharmaceuticals in low- and middle-income countries underscores the need to strengthen drug regulation and post-market surveillance [72].

Effective malaria treatment relies on accurate and timely diagnosis. Conventional microscopy-based diagnosis, while reliable, is labor-intensive and may not be feasible in resource-limited settings. RDTs have been instrumental in improving access to diagnostics, but they have limitations, including the potential for false-negative results and difficulty in detecting low-level infections. Furthermore, parasites have developed deletion of histidine-rich protein, the target proteins in RDTs [12]. The deployment of new highly sensitive RDTs will ensure effective diagnosis and treatment of malaria [73]. Effective combating of malaria also requires addressing the social determinants of health to ensure equitable access to treatment for all. However, low socioeconomic status especially in developing countries, including poverty and lack of education, can exacerbate malaria treatment challenges. Poor communities may face financial barriers in accessing healthcare services and purchasing antimalarial medications. ACTs are generally more expensive than older antimalarial drugs, which can present a barrier to their widespread implementation in resource-limited settings. Furthermore, emerging diseases such as COVID-19 affect the supply and distribution of malaria consumables including medicines and diagnostics. International collaborations and funding initiatives are needed to increase access and affordability.

6. Conclusion

Artemisinin-based combination therapies (ACTs) are safer and remain to be key for malaria control and elimination strategies. DHP and primaquine are promising options for malaria elimination strategies. Malaria treatment faces numerous challenges, from drug resistance to healthcare access limitations and diagnostic difficulties. Addressing these challenges requires a multi-pronged approach, including the development of new antimalarial drugs, strengthening healthcare systems in endemic regions, enhancing diagnostic capabilities, and addressing social and environmental determinants of malaria. Collaboration among governments, international organizations, researchers, and communities is essential to overcome these challenges and ultimately achieve the goal of malaria elimination, improving the health and well-being of millions worldwide.

Conflict of interest

The author declares no conflict of interest.

Notes/thanks/other declarations

NA

DOI: http://dx.doi.org/10.5772/intechopen.113194

Author details

Eulambius Mathias Mlugu
Muhimbili University of Health and Allied Sciences, Dar es Salaam, Tanzania

*Address all correspondence to: mlugusonlove@gmail.com

IntechOpen

© 2023 The Author(s). Licensee IntechOpen. This chapter is distributed under the terms of the Creative Commons Attribution License (http://creativecommons.org/licenses/by/3.0), which permits unrestricted use, distribution, and reproduction in any medium, provided the original work is properly cited.

References

[1] Cowman AF et al. Malaria: Biology and disease. Cell. 2016;**167**:610-624

[2] Feachem RGA et al. Malaria eradication within a generation: Ambitious, achievable, and necessary. Lancet. 2019;**394**(10203):1056-1112

[3] WHO. WHO Global Technical Strategy for Malaria 2016-2030. 2015. Available from: https://reliefweb.int/report/world/who-global-technical-strategy-malaria-2016-2030-2021-update

[4] Haakenstad A et al. Tracking spending on malaria by source in 106 countries, 2000-16: An economic modelling study. The Lancet Infectious Diseases. 2019;**19**:703-716

[5] WHO. World Malaria Report 2022. 2022. Available from: https://www.who.int/teams/global-malaria-programme/reports/world-malaria-report-2022

[6] Ma N et al. The birth of artemisinin. Pharmacology & Therapeutics. 2020;**216**:107658

[7] World Health, O. Guidelines for the Treatment of Malaria. 3rd ed. Geneva: World Health Organization; 2015

[8] Zanghi G, Vaughan AM. Plasmodium vivax pre-erythrocytic stages and the latent hypnozoite. Parasitology International. 2021;**85**:102447

[9] Llanos-Cuentas A et al. Tafenoquine versus primaquine to prevent relapse of Plasmodium vivax malaria. The New England Journal of Medicine. 2019;**380**:229-241

[10] van der Pluijm RW, Imwong M, Chau NH, et al. Determinants of dihydroartemisinin-piperaquine treatment failure in Plasmodium falciparum malaria in Cambodia, Thailand, and Vietnam: A prospective clinical, pharmacological, and genetic study. The Lancet Infectious Diseases. 2019;**19**:952-961

[11] Yimam Y, Mohebali M, Abbaszadeh Afshar MJ. Comparison of diagnostic performance between conventional and ultrasensitive rapid diagnostic tests for diagnosis of malaria: A systematic review and meta-analysis. PLoS One. 2022;**17**:e0263770

[12] Gendrot M et al. Genetic diversity and deletion of Plasmodium falciparum histidine-rich protein 2 and 3: A threat to diagnosis of P. falciparum malaria. Clinical Microbiology and Infection. 2019;**25**:580-585

[13] Arya A et al. Artemisinin-based combination therapy (ACT) and drug resistance molecular markers: A systematic review of clinical studies from two malaria endemic regions-India and sub-Saharan Africa. International Journal for Parasitology: Drugs and Drug Resistance. 2021;**15**:43-56

[14] Frosch AE, Venkatesan M, Laufer MK. Patterns of chloroquine use and resistance in sub-Saharan Africa: A systematic review of household survey and molecular data. Malaria Journal. 2011;**10**:116

[15] van Eijk AM et al. Effect of Plasmodium falciparum sulfadoxine-pyrimethamine resistance on the effectiveness of intermittent preventive therapy for malaria in pregnancy in Africa: A systematic review and meta-analysis. The Lancet Infectious Diseases. 2019;**19**:546-556

[16] WHO. Guideline for the Ttreatment of Malaria. 1st ed2006.

Available from: https://infonet-biovision.org/sites/default/files/1571.treatmentguidelines20061.pdf

[17] Zou Y et al. The effect of artemisinin-based drugs vs non-artemisinin-based drugs on gametophyte carrying in the body after the treatment of uncomplicated falciparum malaria: A systematic review and meta-analysis. Frontiers in Pharmacology. 2021;**12**:707498

[18] Commons RJ et al. The efficacy of dihydroartemisinin-piperaquine and artemether-lumefantrine with and without primaquine on Plasmodium vivax recurrence: A systematic review and individual patient data meta-analysis. PLoS Medicine. 2019;**16**:e1002928

[19] WHO. Global Database on Antimalarial Drug Efficacy and Resistance. 2021. Available from: https://www.who.int/teams/global-malaria-programme/case-management/drug-efficacy-and-resistance/antimalarial-drug-efficacy-database

[20] Cui L, Su XZ. Discovery, mechanisms of action and combination therapy of artemisinin. Expert Review of Anti-Infective Therapy. 2009;**7**:999-1013

[21] Krugliak M, Zhang J, Ginsburg H. Intraerythrocytic Plasmodium falciparum utilizes only a fraction of the amino acids derived from the digestion of host cell cytosol for the biosynthesis of its proteins. Molecular and Biochemical Parasitology. 2002;**119**:249-256

[22] Sibley CH et al. Pyrimethamine-sulfadoxine resistance in Plasmodium falciparum: What next? Trends in Parasitology. 2001;**17**:582-588

[23] Nzila A et al. Comparative folate metabolism in humans and malaria parasites (part I): Pointers for malaria treatment from cancer chemotherapy. Trends in Parasitology. 2005;**21**:292-298

[24] WHO. Artemether-Lumefantrine Summary of Product Characteristics. Available from: https://extranet.who.int/pqweb/sites/default/files/MA120part4.pdf

[25] Abdulla S, Sagara I. Dispersible formulation of artemether/lumefantrine: Specifically developed for infants and young children. Malaria Journal. 2009;**8**(Suppl 1):S7

[26] Shibeshi W et al. Efficacy and safety of artemisinin-based combination therapy for the treatment of uncomplicated malaria in pregnant women: A systematic review and meta-analysis. Therapeutics and Clinical Risk Management. 2021;**17**:1353-1370

[27] WHO. Dihydroartemisinin-Piperaquine Summary of Product Characteristics. Available from: https://extranet.who.int/pqweb/sites/default/files/MA139part4v11_0.pdf

[28] WHO. Artesunate-Amodiaquine Summary of Product Characteristics. Available from: https://extranet.who.int/pqweb/sites/default/files/documents/MA081part4v1.pdf

[29] WHO. Artesunate-Mefloquine Summary of Product Characteristics. Available from: https://extranet.who.int/pqweb/sites/default/files/MA078part4v2.pdf

[30] WHO. Artesunate-Pyronaridine Summary of Product Characteristics. Available from: https://www.ema.europa.eu/en/documents/outside-eu-product-information/pyramax-product-information_en.pdf

[31] WHO. Chloroquine Summary of Product Characteristics. Available from:

https://www.medicines.org.uk/emc/product/5490/smpc/print

[32] Stepniewska K et al. Safety of single-dose primaquine as a Plasmodium falciparum gametocytocide: A systematic review and meta-analysis of individual patient data. BMC Medicine. 2022;**20**:350

[33] Marwa K, Kapesa A, Baraka V, Konje E, Kidenya B, et al. Therapeutic efficacy of artemether-lumefantrine, artesunate-amodiaquine and dihydroartemisinin-piperaquine in the treatment of uncomplicated *Plasmodium falciparum* malaria in sub-Saharan Africa: A systematic review and meta-analysis. PLoS One. 2022;**17**(3):e0264339

[34] Cubillos AL, Porras A, Rico A. Efficacy of tafenoquine in the prophylaxis and treatment of malaria by Plasmodium vivax, systematic review and meta-analysis. Biomédica. 2022;**42**:364-377

[35] Mwaiswelo RO et al. A single low dose of primaquine is safe and sufficient to reduce transmission of Plasmodium falciparum gametocytes regardless of cytochrome P450 2D6 enzyme activity in Bagamoyo district, Tanzania. Malaria Journal. 2022;**21**:84

[36] Nelwan EJ, Shakinah S, Pasaribu A. Association of G6PD status and haemolytic anaemia in patients receiving anti-malarial agents: A systematic review and meta-analysis. Malaria Journal. 2023;**22**(1):77

[37] White NJ. Anaemia and malaria. Malaria Journal. 2018;**17**:371

[38] Song X et al. Cerebral malaria induced by Plasmodium falciparum: Clinical features, pathogenesis, diagnosis, and treatment. Frontiers in Cellular and Infection Microbiology. 2022;**12**:939532

[39] WHO. Methods for Surveillance of Antimalarial Drug Efficacy. 2009. Available from: https://www.who.int/publications/i/item/9789241597531

[40] Shibeshi W et al. Efficacy and safety of artemisinin-based combination therapies for the treatment of uncomplicated malaria in pediatrics: A systematic review and meta-analysis. BMC Infectious Diseases. 2021;**21**:326

[41] Ashley EA, Dhorda M, Fairhurst RM, Amaratunga C, Lim P, Suon S, et al.; Tracking Resistance to Artemisinin Collaboration (TRAC). Spread of artemisinin resistance in Plasmodium falciparum malaria. The New England Journal of Medicine. 2014;**371**(5):411-423

[42] Price RN, von Seidlein L, Valecha N, Nosten F, Baird JK, White NJ. Global extent of chloroquine-resistant Plasmodium vivax: A systematic review and meta-analysis. The Lancet Infectious Diseases. 2014;**14**(10):982-991

[43] Ross LS, Fidock DA. Elucidating mechanisms of drug-resistant Plasmodium falciparum. Cell Host & Microbe. 2019;**26**(1):35-47

[44] Phyo AP, Ashley EA, Anderson TJC, Bozdech Z, Carrara VI, Sriprawat K, et al. Declining efficacy of artemisinin combination therapy against P. falciparum malaria on the Thai-Myanmar border (2003-2013): The role of parasite genetic factors. Clinical Infectious Diseases. 2016;**63**(6):784-791. DOI: 10.1093/cid/ciw388

[45] Juma DW, Omondi AA, Ingasia L, Opot B, Cheruiyot A, Yeda R, et al. Trends in drug resistance codons in Plasmodium falciparum dihydrofolate reductase and dihydropteroate synthase genes in Kenyan parasites from 2008 to 2012. Malaria Journal. 2014;**13**:250

[46] Desai M, Gutman J, Taylor SM, Wiegand RE, Khairallah C, Kayentao K, et al. Impact of sulfadoxine-pyrimethamine resistance on effectiveness of intermittent preventive therapy for malaria in pregnancy at clearing infections and preventing low birth weight. Clinical Infectious Diseases. 2016;**62**:323-333

[47] Bassi PU et al. Cohort event monitoring of patients treated for uncomplicated malaria with artemisinin-based combination therapies in selected hospitals and community pharmacies in Nigeria. The Nigerian Postgraduate Medical Journal. 2016;**23**:172-181

[48] Bakshi R et al. An integrated assessment of the clinical safety of artemether-lumefantrine: A new oral fixed-dose combination antimalarial drug. Transactions of the Royal Society of Tropical Medicine and Hygiene. 2000;**94**:419-424

[49] Funck-Brentano C et al. Evaluation of the effects on the QT-interval of 4 artemisinin-based combination therapies with a correction-free and heart rate-free method. Scientific Reports. 2019;**9**:883

[50] Chan XHS et al. Risk of sudden unexplained death after use of dihydroartemisinin-piperaquine for malaria: A systematic review and Bayesian meta-analysis. The Lancet Infectious Diseases. 2018;**18**:913-923

[51] Assefa DG et al. Safety of dihydroartemisinin-piperaquine versus artemether-lumefantrine for the treatment of uncomplicated Plasmodium falciparum malaria among children in Africa: A systematic review and meta-analysis of randomized control trials. Malaria Journal. 2022;**21**:4

[52] Salanti A et al. Evidence for the involvement of VAR2CSA in pregnancy-associated malaria. The Journal of Experimental Medicine. 2004;**200**:1197-1203

[53] Mlugu EM et al. Prevalence and correlates of asymptomatic malaria and anemia on first antenatal care visit among pregnant women in southeast, Tanzania. International Journal of Environmental Research and Public Health. 2020;**17**:3123

[54] Briand V et al. Intermittent preventive treatment for the prevention of malaria during pregnancy in high transmission areas. Malaria Journal. 2007;**6**:160

[55] Mlugu EM et al. Effectiveness of sulfadoxine-pyrimethamine for intermittent preventive treatment of malaria and adverse birth outcomes in pregnant women. Pathogens. 2020;**9**:207

[56] Waltmann A et al. The positive effect of malaria IPTp-SP on birthweight is mediated by gestational weight gain but modifiable by maternal carriage of enteric pathogens. eBioMedicine. 2022;**77**:103871

[57] Mlugu EM et al. Effectiveness of intermittent preventive treatment with dihydroartemisinin-piperaqunine against malaria in pregnancy in Tanzania: A randomized controlled trial. Clinical Pharmacology and Therapeutics. 2021;**110**:1478-1489

[58] WHO. World Malaria Report 2022. Available from: https://www.who.int/publications/i/item/9789240064898 [Accessed: May 18, 2023]

[59] Mwaiswelo RO, Mmbando BP, Chacky F, Molteni F, Mohamed A, Lazaro S, et al. Malaria infection and anemia status in under-five children from southern Tanzania where seasonal malaria chemoprevention is being implemented. PLoS One. 2021;**16**(12):e0260785

[60] Dabira ED et al. Mass drug administration of ivermectin and dihydroartemisinin-piperaquine against malaria in settings with high coverage of standard control interventions: A cluster-randomised controlled trial in the Gambia. The Lancet Infectious Diseases. 2022;**22**:519-528

[61] Shah MP et al. Mass drug administration for malaria. Cochrane Database of Systematic Reviews. 2021;**9**:Cd008846

[62] Reuter SE et al. Effect of food on the pharmacokinetics of piperaquine and dihydroartemisinin. Clinical Drug Investigation. 2015;**35**:559-567

[63] Borrmann S et al. The effect of food consumption on lumefantrine bioavailability in African children receiving artemether-lumefantrine crushed or dispersible tablets (Coartem) for acute uncomplicated Plasmodium falciparum malaria. Tropical Medicine & International Health. 2010;**15**:434-441

[64] Staehli Hodel EM et al. Effect of single nucleotide polymorphisms in cytochrome P450 isoenzyme and N-acetyltransferase 2 genes on the metabolism of artemisinin-based combination therapies in malaria patients from Cambodia and Tanzania. Antimicrobial Agents and Chemotherapy. 2013;**57**:950-958

[65] Mutagonda RF et al. Pregnancy and CYP3A5 genotype affect day 7 plasma lumefantrine concentrations. Drug Metabolism and Disposition. 2019;**47**:1415-1424

[66] Duru V, Witkowski B, Ménard D. Plasmodium falciparum resistance to artemisinin derivatives and piperaquine: A major challenge for malaria elimination in Cambodia. The American Journal of Tropical Medicine and Hygiene. 2016;**95**:1228-1238

[67] de Haan F et al. Expert perspectives on the introduction of triple artemisinin-based combination therapies (TACTs) in southeast Asia: A delphi study. BMC Public Health. 2022;**22**:864

[68] Mlugu EM et al. Pregnancy increases CYP3A enzymes activity as measured by the 4β-hydroxycholesterol/cholesterol ratio. International Journal of Molecular Sciences. 2022;**23**:15168

[69] WorldWide Antimalarial Resistance Network (WWARN) Lumefantrine PK/PD Study Group. Artemether-lumefantrine treatment of uncomplicated Plasmodium falciparum malaria: A systematic review and meta-analysis of day 7 lumefantrine concentrations and therapeutic response using individual patient data. BMC Medicine. 2015;**13**:227

[70] Kloprogge F et al. Artemether-lumefantrine dosing for malaria treatment in young children and pregnant women: A pharmacokinetic-pharmacodynamic meta-analysis. PLoS Medicine. 2018;**15**:e1002579

[71] Ozawa S et al. Prevalence and estimated economic burden of substandard and falsified medicines in low- and middle-income countries: A systematic review and meta-analysis. JAMA Network Open. 2018;**1**:e181662

[72] Newton PN, Bond KC. Global access to quality-assured medical products: The Oxford statement and call to action. The Lancet Global Health. 2019;**7**:e1609-e1611

[73] Slater HC et al. Performance and utility of more highly sensitive malaria rapid diagnostic tests. BMC Infectious Diseases. 2022;**22**:121

Chapter 8

Antimalarial Drugs with Quinoline Nucleus and Analogs

Deto Ursul Jean-Paul N'guessan, Songuigama Coulibaly, Apleheni Eunice Melissa Adouko and Mahama Ouattara

Abstract

Quinoline core antimalarials are a major class used for the management of uncomplicated malaria in combination with artemisinin derivatives. Moreover, despite its adverse effects, Quinine remains the reference molecule in the treatment of cerebral malaria due to *Plasmodium falciparum*. This class also contains molecules such as Mefloquine used in the prevention of malaria. In addition, synthetic derivatives are more manageable with greater therapeutic margins and fewer adverse effects. They have an interest in avoiding the spread of resistance, especially with derivatives possessing gametocytocidal activities. With the presence of a chloroquine-resistant strain of *Plasmodium*, the use of synthetic derivatives as monotherapy is prohibited to avoid the spread of resistance in this class. In this chapter, we propose to present the class of antimalarials with a quinoline nucleus under its pharmacochemical aspects as well as the prospects for its development to preserve and improve the effectiveness of its representatives in the management of malaria.

Keywords: quinoline, *Plasmodium*, antiprotozoal, antimalarial, chloroquine resistance

1. Introduction

Malaria is one of the deadliest parasitic diseases. Global mortality from this disease has increased in recent years due to the impact of Covid-19. Indeed, since 2020, the WHO has reported more than 600,000 deaths each year, the majority of which occur in Africa and tropical regions [1]. This mosquito-borne parasitosis affects millions of people each year, with significant socio-economic consequences [2].

The therapeutic arsenal used to prevent and treat malaria mainly comprises, on the one hand, antimalarials with a quinoline nucleus and, on the other hand, artemisinin and its derivatives. All antimalarials work by interfering with the life cycle of plasmodium in the human body. They can target different stages of the parasite cycle, such as the reproduction of the parasite in the red blood cells, they are called erythrocytes schizonticides or their development in the liver, in the case of tissue schizonticides.

IntechOpen

Antimalarial drugs with quinoline patterns and analogs constitute a homogeneous class of antiparasitic-antiprotozoal drugs. They are mostly of natural or synthetic origin. They proceed by blocking the growth of parasites of the genus *Plasmodium*, the causative agents of paludism or Malaria. They are used in the treatment of uncomplicated malaria and severe malaria. Quinine is an essential drug for the treatment of cerebral malaria because truly little resistance has been reported [2, 3].

From the point of view of their chemical constitution, they all have in their respective molecules the quinoline nucleus or a similar tricyclic unit.

Over time, the malaria parasite has developed resistance to certain antimalarials, in this case chloroquine. This has led to the appearance and proliferation of chloroquine-resistant strains of Plasmodium [4, 5]. This resistance has limited the effectiveness of these drugs in certain regions of the world, forcing the development of new therapeutic options.

Thus, the challenge for pharmacochemists has been to develop effective antimalarials on these resistant strains and to protect their effectiveness, in particular by drug combinations.

Finding effective treatments for malaria is therefore a global public health priority.

Understanding the chemistry and pharmacology of this class of drugs is essential to improving their efficacy and developing new therapeutic agents.

This chapter aims on the one hand to present the chemical aspects of quinoline core antimalarial drugs and their structural analogs; and on the other hand, to highlight the link that exists between the structural elements and their mechanisms of action or even their therapeutic implications, justifying their current use in the treatment of malaria.

2. Natural prototype: quinine

2.1 Structure and origin

2.1.1 Structure

Quinine is a 4-methanol quinoline derivative. It is characterized by the presence of four asymmetric carbons in its structure. Therefore, two forms are distinguished: the levogyre form and the dextrorotatory form. Only the levogyre form (quinine, **Figure 1**) has antimalarial properties. The dextrorotatory form (quinidine) has essentially antiarrhythmic properties. Quinine and quinidine are distinguished from each other based on methanolic carbon stereochemistry [2, 3].

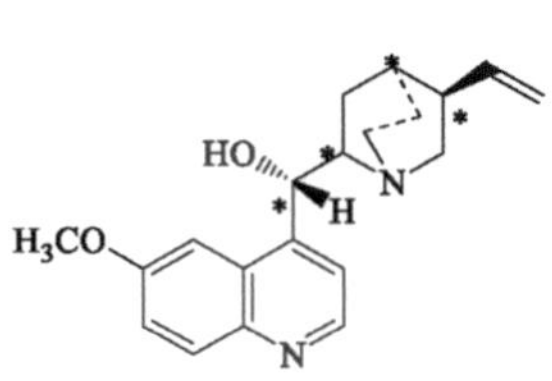

Figure 1.
Quinine (Quinimax ®).

Quinine has a heterocyclic structure comprising four rings, two of which are aromatic in nature at the quinoline level and two in the bicyclic amine called quinuclidine. The presence of these rings gives quinine good hydrophobicity.

2.1.2 Origin

Quinine is an alkaloid extracted with quinidine, Cinchonine and Cinchonidine from cinchona bark of Peru in the form of sulfate. For the other salts: Quinine base released by treatment with NaOH then salified (Hydrohydrate, formate) [2, 6, 7].

2.2 Spectrum of action and limits of use

2.2.1 Action spectrum

Specificity: Quinine primarily targets the erythrocytic stage of the malaria parasite's life cycle and may not be effective against other stages (such as the liver stage). It is a fast-acting erythrocytic schizontocide acting on the endoerythrocytic forms of all Plasmodium species (*P. falciparum, P. vivax, P. malariae* and *P ovale*). However, it is inactive on mature gametocytes of *P. falciparum* [2, 6].

2.2.2 Usage limits

- Limitation

The synthesis of quinine is long and expensive. Thus, it is not very profitable, so the quinine marketed is mainly extractive origin.

Quinine has a narrow therapeutic window. Indeed, the effective plasma concentration is between 2 and 5 μg/ml. In addition, the toxic concentration is around 7 μg/ml. Hence, the need to repeat the doses three times a day [8–11].

- Side effects

Quinine is an antimalarial drug with a long history of use. While it has been effective in treating malaria, it does have limitations and side effects, here are some of the associated aspects:

The most common side effects are:

- Gastrointestinal effects: this drug can cause nausea, vomiting, and abdominal pain.
- Cardiovascular effects: Quinine has been associated with cardiac arrhythmias and can have negative effects on the heart, especially when administered intravenously in high doses.
- Cinchonism: Quinine can cause a condition called cinchonism, characterized by symptoms such as tinnitus (ringing in the ears), headache, dizziness, and visual disturbances.

- Retinopathy: Prolonged use of chloroquine, particularly at high doses, may lead to retinopathy, which can affect vision [6].

- Reasons that led to the development of synthesis derivatives to overcome these drawbacks

The development of synthetic derivatives of antimalarial drugs was driven by several reasons, including the need to overcome limitations and improve the therapeutic properties of existing antimalarials. Here are some key reasons:

- Enhancing efficacy: Many natural antimalarial compounds, such as quinine from the cinchona tree, exhibited therapeutic properties but had limitations in terms of their efficacy. Hemisynthesis and synthesis of derivatives allowed modifications of the chemical structure to enhance the potency and effectiveness against malaria parasites [12–14].

- Overcoming resistance: The emergence of drug resistance in malaria parasites, particularly to drugs like chloroquine, necessitated the development of new compounds. By modifying the chemical structure through hemisynthesis and synthesis, researchers aimed to create derivatives with improved efficacy against drug-resistant strains of the malaria parasite [2, 9, 10].

- Improving safety and tolerability: Some natural antimalarial compounds may have significant side effects or toxicity when used at effective doses. Hemisynthesis and synthesis allowed for the modification of the chemical structure to retain antimalarial activity while reducing adverse effects or improving the drug's safety profile [8, 13].

- Pharmacokinetic properties: Hemisynthesis and synthesis of derivatives also focused on improving the pharmacokinetic properties of antimalarial drugs. This includes factors such as bioavailability, distribution in the body, metabolism, and elimination. Optimization of these properties can enhance the drug's efficacy and patient compliance [4, 14].

By exploring hemisynthesis and synthesis techniques, researchers can modify the chemical structure of natural antimalarial compounds to address these factors, ultimately leading to the development of more effective, safer, and commercially viable antimalarial drugs.

- Key points

Quinine is a natural molecule used in levogyre form.

It has a basic character due to the presence of its nitrogen atoms. This character is used for the preparation of water-soluble salts which can be administered intravenously.

Adverse effects are often dose-dependent. Moreover, the chemical synthesis of quinine is difficult and expensive. Hence the need to develop synthetic derivatives [2, 3, 6, 7].

3. Synthetic derivatives

This part is dedicated to the presentation of the different classes of quinoline antimalarial drugs according to their chemical structure.

3.1 Classification

Quinoline antimalarial drugs can be classified into several categories according to their chemical structure.

This classification is based on substituents on quinoline and the number of cycles. Indeed, there are four chemical series:

- 4-methanol quinolines (**Figure 2**)
- 4-amino quinolines (**Figure 3**)
- 8-amino quinolines (**Figure 4**)
- Tricyclic analogs (**Figure 5**)

3.2 Structures

Here are some of the major classes of quinoline antimalarial drugs and some examples of drugs in each class [3, 6–8, 15].

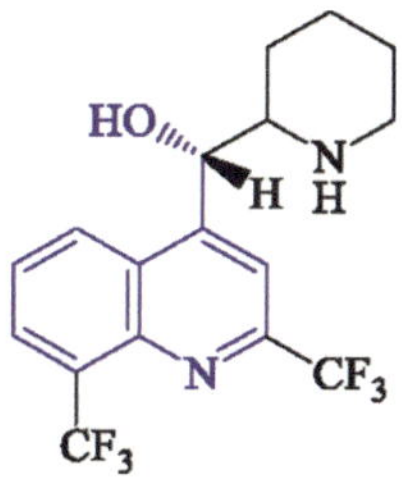

Figure 2.
Méfloquine (Lariam ®).

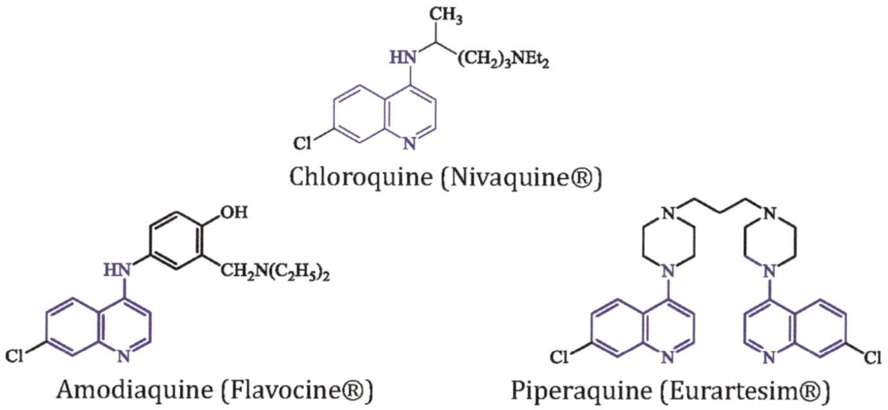

Figure 3.
4-Aminoquinolines antimalarial.

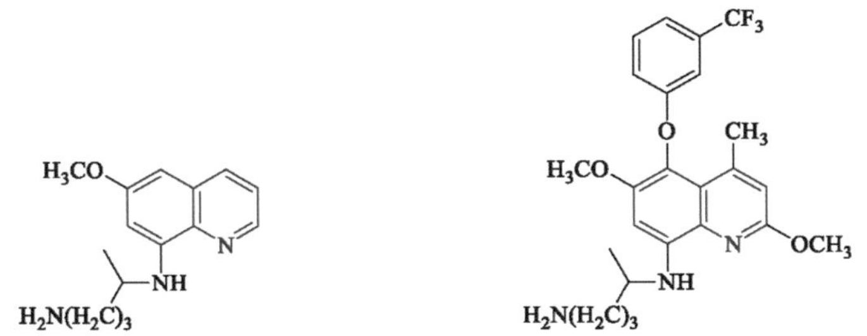

Primaquine (Primaquine®) Tafenoquine (Krintafel®)

Figure 4.
8-Aminoquinolines antimalarial.

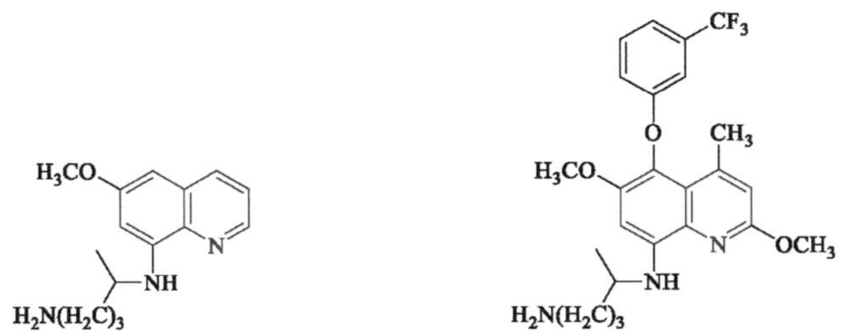

- Primaquine (Primaquine®) Tafenoquine (Krintafel®)

Figure 5.
Antimalarial agents with tricyclic nucleus.

3.2.1 4-Methanol quinolines

Mefloquine is a synthetic quinoline attached to a piperidine ring at the level of the methanolic chain at 4. In addition, we note the presence of two trifluoromethyl groups on the quinoline in position 2 and 8. All these ring and substituents make it possible to preserve the lipophilicity of the molecule.

3.2.2 4-Aminoquinolines

Chloroquine is an aminoquinoline derivative with an aliphatic diethylamine side chain on the amine at position 4. Amodiaquine has in its structure a diaminoalkyl side chain with a phenolic group. Piperaquine is a bisquinoline whose linker chain on the amines in position 4 has two piperazines.

3.2.3 8-Aminoquinolines

Tafenoquine (**Figure 4**) is a prodrug whose active form, obtained after metabolization, is quinone Tafenoquine. Primaquine has a Quinoline nucleus carrying a methoxyl group at 6 like quinine and an amine at 8. The side chain on this amine is aliphatic in nature with a terminal primary amine. Tafenoquine is distinguished by the presence in position 5 of the quinoline, a phenolic group carrying a trifluoromethyl.

3.2.4 Tricyclic analogs

- Lumefantrine (**Figure 5**) is a derivative with a fluorene nucleus, while pyronaridine is a 8-Azaacridine's derivative. Pyronaridine (**Figure 5**) is actually a 4-aminoquinoline fused to a pyridine. The side chain on the amine carries a phenolic ring doubly substituted by a methyl pyrrolidine chain. Lumefantrine is a synthetic aryl amino-alcohol compound that is structurally related to chloroquine by the presence of a butylamine chain [6, 15, 16].

4. Pharmacochemical aspects

4.1 Mechanism of action

8-Aminoquinolines, such as primaquine and tafenoquine, act primarily against the hypnozoite (dormant) forms of the *Plasmodium* parasite in the liver, making them particularly effective against the latent form of malaria caused by *Plasmodium vivax* and *Plasmodium ovale* [8, 12].

The precise mechanism of action of 8-aminoquinolines is not fully understood, but they are thought to interfere with the metabolism of heme, a molecule essential for parasite survival. 8-Aminoquinolines cause toxic heme buildup in parasites, which leads to oxidative damage and parasite death [12].

In contrast, other classes of antimalarials with a quinoline core, such as 4-aminoquinolines and quinine, have a different mechanism of action. They act primarily by inhibiting the polymerization of heme to hematozin, which leads to toxic accumulation of free heme in the parasites. This disrupts the metabolism of the parasite and ultimately leads to its death [8, 9].

4.2 Pharmacotherapeutic activity of the quinolines antimalarial

This chapter presents the exploration of the relationship between the chemical structure of quinoline antimalarial drugs and their pharmacological activity. The relationship between the chemical structure of quinoline antimalarial drugs and their pharmacological activity is complex and multifaceted. However, there are some general structural features that contribute to their antimalarial activity [2, 5, 7, 8, 12, 16]. Here are some key aspects.

4.2.1 Indispensable structural elements

- Quinoline core (**Figure 6**): Quinoline is a heterocyclic aromatic compound that forms the core structure of many antimalarial drugs, such as chloroquine and quinine.

Quinine works by binding to 18S ribosomal RNA, which is essential for parasite protein synthesis. This interaction disrupts the function of ribosomal RNA, thus inhibiting the normal protein synthesis of the parasite and leading to its death [2, 8, 17].

More specifically, the quinoline core of quinine is involved in π-π interactions with specific nucleotide bases of 18S ribosomal RNA. These π-π interactions involve the pi (π) electrons from the aromatic rings of the quinoline nucleus and the pi (π) electrons

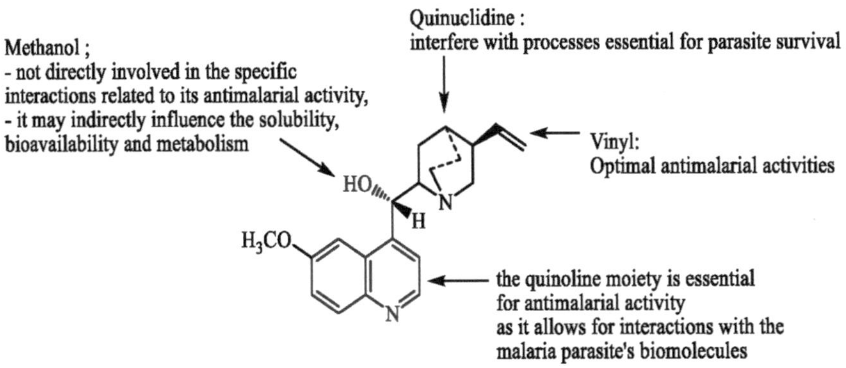

Figure 6.
Summary of SAR of quinine.

from the nucleotide bases of RNA. This pi-π bond stabilizes the bond between quinine and ribosomal RNA, thus promoting the inhibition of protein synthesis [2, 8, 16].

Additionally, the quinoline core of quinine can form hydrogen bonds with specific residues of ribosomal RNA, thereby enhancing the ligand-receptor interaction [2, 8, 16].

- The vinyl group (**Figure 6**) and the quinuclidine ring of quinine play a key role by causing its antimalarial activities. The vinyl group is involved in interactions with the ion channels of the parasite, while the quinuclidine ring allows binding to specific proteins or receptors of the parasite. The stereochemistry of the quinuclidine ring is also important for quinine activity. In fact, the vinyl group, allows quinine to interact with specific cellular targets of the malaria parasite, such as the ion channels present in the membranes of the parasite. These interactions can disrupt ion flow and other vital processes within the parasite, leading to its death or inability to grow and reproduce [6].

- The quinuclidine ring (**Figure 6**), which is a cyclic structure containing a nitrogen atom, also confers antimalarial properties to quinine. This structure is important for the binding of quinine to certain specific parasite proteins or receptors. For example, quinuclidine can bind to parasite proteins involved in ion transport, pH regulation, and other processes essential for parasite survival. Furthermore, the quinuclidine ring of quinine also contributes to its stereochemistry, which means that its spatial configuration is important for its antimalarial activity. Studies have shown that the specific configuration of certain atoms in the quinuclidine ring is crucial for the interaction of quinine with its cellular targets and for its antimalarial efficacy [6, 13].

- The methanol group (**Figure 6**) is a substituent present in the structure of quinine. It is not directly involved in the specific interactions between quinine and the cellular targets of the malaria parasite. These interactions are mainly mediated by other parts of the quinine molecule, such as the quinuclidine ring and the vinyl group [6, 13].

However, the presence of the methanol group can have an impact on the solubility of quinine in biological solvents and pharmaceutical formulations. Good solubility of quinine is essential so that it can be well absorbed in the body after administration and reach the desired sites of action. Solubility can also affect the release rate and distribution of quinine in tissues.

Furthermore, the methanol moiety may also be involved in the metabolic reactions of quinine in the body. Quinine undergoes metabolism and elimination processes in the liver and kidneys, and functional groups such as methanol may play a role in these processes [6, 12, 13].

Overall, the presence of four cycles in quinoline and quinuclidine nucleus allows this molecule to increase the hydrophobicity of the molecule as well as good crossing of the blood-brain barrier. This particularity is relevant in the treatment of cerebral malaria [6, 12, 13].

In some national therapeutic protocols for the management of malaria, Quinine by IV infusion is used to manage severe malaria. In pregnant women, Quinine *per os* is used first [12].

4.2.2 4-methanolquinoline series

- Molecular simplification of quinuclidine

The addition of trifluoromethyl groups (**Figure 7**) to mefloquine was carried out with the aim of improving its antimalarial activity and increasing its lipophilicity, which promotes its penetration into cells infected by the parasite responsible for malaria (*Plasmodium*). Trifluoromethyl groups may influence the interaction of mefloquine with its specific cellular targets, such as ion channels, receptors, or enzymes involved in parasite metabolism [6, 12]. It has increased potency against chloroquine-resistant strains of malaria and has a prolonged half-life compared to quinine.

Regarding the potential CNS toxicity of mefloquine, trifluoromethyl groups may play a role in this property. Mefloquine can cross the blood-brain barrier and bind to receptors in the brain, which can cause neurological side effects in some individuals. Trifluoromethyl groups can influence the affinity of mefloquine for these receptors and thus modulate its effect on the central nervous system [6, 12, 13].

4.2.3 Aminoquinolines

Aminoquinoline derivatives, such as chloroquine and amodiaquine, have an amino group attached to the quinoline ring. This amino group is thought to be crucial for the drugs' antimalarial activity. It helps in the accumulation of the drug within the parasite's acidic digestive vacuole, disrupting its physiological processes [12, 13].

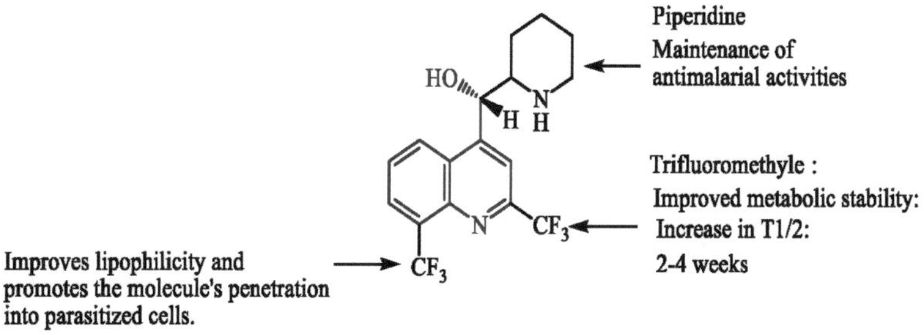

Figure 7.
Summary of SAR of mefloquine.

- The chlorine atom of chloroquine (**Figure 8**) is responsible for several key interactions with the biological target, namely the malaria parasite. These interactions are mainly mediated by chemical bonds and intermolecular forces between chlorine and the specific components of the parasite [6, 13].

- More precisely, the chlorine atom of chloroquine is involved in interactions with the nucleic acid of the parasite, in particular DNA. It binds to nucleobases, thereby disrupting the structure and function of parasitic DNA. This DNA disruption leads to damage at the genetic level, preventing the replication of the parasite and ultimately leading to its death [6].

- In addition, the chlorine atom of chloroquine can also interact with other cellular components of the parasite, such as proteins essential for its survival. These additional interactions contribute to the effectiveness of chloroquine as an antimalarial agent [12, 13].

It should be noted that the precise mechanisms by which chloroquine interacts with *Plasmodium* are complex and are still the subject of extensive research. However, it is well established that the presence of the chlorine atom in the structure of chloroquine is crucial for its antimalarial activity by specifically targeting the parasite and disrupting its vital processes [6, 12, 13].

- Basicity and ionization: The basicity of the nitrogen atom in the quinoline ring in chloroquine affects the molecule's ability to interact with acidic compartments, including the nutrient vacuole of the malaria parasite. Indeed, it is an antimalarial with a quinoline nucleus having a weak base character, allowing the trapping of ions in the acid vacuole of the parasite and preventing the phenomenon of efflux [6, 12, 13].

- The tertiary amine of the diamino alkyl chain gives chloroquine basic properties, which facilitates its diffusion through the cell membranes of the parasite when it is in non-ionized form. Moreover, in ionized form under the acidic conditions of the food vacuole, this tertiary amine plays a crucial role in the inhibition of the formation of β-hematin by ionic interaction and in the accumulation of the molecule within *Plasmodium* [6, 12, 13].

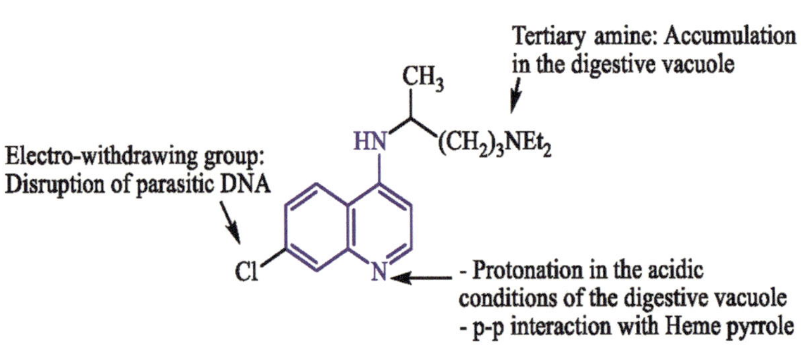

Figure 8.
Summary of SAR of chloroquine.

The main limit of the use of chloroquine was the appearance and development of resistance in many parts of the world, particularly in areas with high levels of malaria transmission. *Plasmodium falciparum* strains with mutations in the chloroquine target protein, known as *P. falciparum chloroquine* resistance transporter (PfCRT), are less susceptible to the drug's action [2, 9–11].

In short, the first two molecules obtained by pharmacomodulation of the basic structure of Quinine with the aim of having on the one hand molecules of easy chemical access, and on the other hand more manageable molecules with a wide therapeutic margin were Mefloquine and Chloroquine [2].

Indeed, it appeared that Mefloquine exhibited increased neurotoxicity, and a long half-life and was sold at a high cost. This led to the decline of the 4-methanol-quinoline series [2].

Chloroquine was less toxic than Quinine. However, the emergence of chloroquine drug-resistant *P. falciparum* has also shown the limit of this series of 4-aminoquinolines. Thus, other pharmacomodulations were undertaken in this last series, with the aim of improving antimalarial activity on gametocytes, intrahepatic forms and reducing toxicity [2, 11].

Since then, two main modulations have been undertaken by pharmacochemists on the structure of chloroquine. One at the diaminoalkyl chain, the other at the position of the amine function.

4.3 Structural modifications of the quinoline structures and its antimalaria potency

Structural modifications have been made to chloroquine to improve its antimalarial activity against resistant strains or enhance its pharmacokinetic properties. Here are some examples.

4.3.1 Incorporation of an aromatic ring into the diaminoalkyl chain

The introduction of side chain modifications of chloroquine may enhance its antimalarial activity. Indeed, the cyclization of the butyl side chain to a phenyl-like aryl chain results in the synthesis of Amodiaquine, which exhibits increased potency against resistant strains of malaria. In addition, this derivative also has a reduced toxicity compared to chloroquine [4, 16].

4.3.2 Changing the length of the aminoalkyl chain

The incorporation of the nitrogen of the aminoalkyl chain in a piperazine cycle, associated with the duplication of the 7-chloroquinoline motif, led to the production of Piperaquine.

Piperaquine (**Figure 3**) is a bisquinoline derivative containing two quinoline rings linked by a piperazine linker. The presence of its six nitrogen atoms, would allow a better accumulation in the digestive vacuole by protonation. It has improved pharmacokinetic properties and is effective against chloroquine-resistant strains due to its stability against efflux [16].

4.3.3 Displacement of the diaminoalkyl chain in position 8

Primaquine (**Figure 9**) is an 8-aminoquinoline derivative, currently used for the treatment of *Plasmodium vivax* and *Plasmodium ovale* malaria. Interestingly, it is

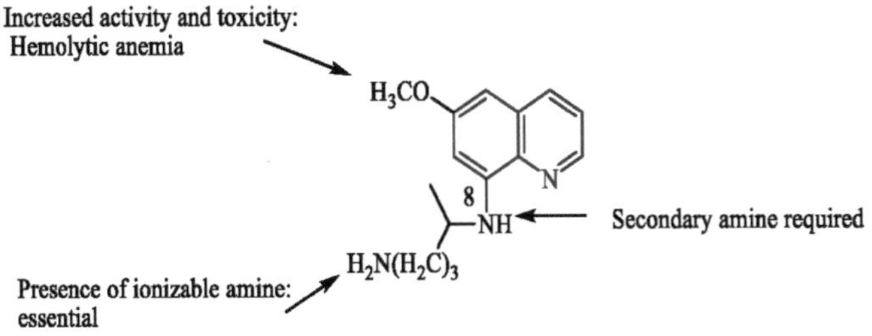

Figure 9.
Summary of SAR on primaquine.

active on *Plasmodium falciparum* gametocytes and active on hepatic hypnozoite forms and has been used for malarial prophylaxis [4, 16].

Tafenoquine is structurally related to primaquine and is approved for the prevention of relapse of *Plasmodium vivax* malaria, when co-administered with chloroquine. It exhibits potent activity against *Plasmodium vivax* and *Plasmodium falciparum*, including drug-resistant strains. Tafenoquine has a long half-life, allowing for a single-dose treatment option [4, 16].

4.3.4 Isosteric replacements

Replacing the quinoline ring with tricyclic isosteres such as a pyridoquinoline (Aza-acridine) or fluorene ring in compounds like pyronaridine and lumefantrine (**Figure 5**) has led to increased antimalarial activity. The presence of these isosteric nuclei gives these molecules special features in terms of their mechanism of action [2, 4, 13, 16, 18].

- The pyronaridine is an aminoalkoxy derivative having an aza-acridine core that would act as a facilitator of pi-pi interactions, helping to block the biopolymerization of β-hematin into hemozoin, and thus facilitating the accumulation of toxic hematin in the digestive vacuole of the parasite [2, 4, 13, 16, 18].

- The fluorene ring of lumefantrine would play a key role by increasing the solubility of the molecule in lipids, which facilitates its incorporation into the membranes of the parasites responsible for malaria. This interaction with parasitic membranes contributes to its accumulation in fatty tissue and prolongs the half-life of lumefantrine to 4–6 days [2, 4, 13, 16, 18].

- The aminoalkyl alcohol side chain of Lumefantrine would have the ability to associate with heme, a hemoglobin degradation molecule. The interaction between lumefantrine and heme disrupts the process of heme degradation, leading to toxic accumulation of heme in the parasite and thus causing its death. This molecule exhibits improved pharmacokinetic properties, such as better absorption and a longer half-life than chloroquine. It is used in combination with artemether as a first-line treatment for uncomplicated malaria [2, 4, 13, 16, 18].

These examples highlight the successful application of structural modifications to the chloroquine scaffold to improve antimalarial activity and overcome drug resistance.

In summary, RSA studies have shown that the quinoline nucleus contributes to the onset and maintenance of antimalarial activity, by contributing to the inhibition of the formation of hemozoin from the heme of parasitized erythrocytes.

The increase in the number of nitrogen atoms will contribute to better activity on resistant Plasmodium strains.

4.4 Principles of combinations of antimalarials based on artemisinin derivatives

Quinoline derivatives have been widely used in combination therapies for the treatment of malaria.

The antimalarial combination refers to the use of two or more antimalarial drugs with different mechanisms of action to treat malaria. This approach is used to improve the effectiveness of treatment, delays the development of drug resistance and improves the speed of remission of patients.

Indeed, when two or more drugs with different mechanisms of action are used together, the likelihood of a parasite acquiring resistance to all drugs simultaneously is greatly reduced. It is thus more difficult for resistant strains to emerge and spread in the population. Artemisinin derivatives have a short half-life, which means they are eliminated quickly from the body. By combining them with quinoline derivative drugs with a longer half-life, the selection pressure on the parasites is reduced, thus limiting the emergence of resistance. In addition, by using combinations, the effectiveness of quinoline drugs can be preserved for a longer time [6, 12].

- Synergistic action: The drugs in the combination work together, enhancing their individual activities and improving overall antimalarial efficacy. Synergy occurs when the combined action of the drugs is greater than the sum of their individual effects. This synergistic interaction can lead to increased parasite killing, faster clearance of the infection, and improved treatment outcomes.

This is the case with artemisinin derivatives. Artemisinin derivatives have a rapid and powerful action against the parasites responsible for malaria. They quickly reduce the parasite load in the blood, which can quickly relieve symptoms and prevent serious complications. By combining quinoline drugs with other antimalarials, the overall efficacy is enhanced by attacking the parasites at different stages of their life cycle, leading to better parasite clearance and improved treatment outcomes. Combination antimalarials have shown higher efficacy in the treatment of uncomplicated malaria compared to monotherapy [6, 12].

- Broadening activity spectrum: Combination therapies can extend coverage against different species of Plasmodium parasites. Certain quinoline derivatives, such as Amodiaquine are effective against certain species like Plasmodium falciparum, while primaquine, is more active against Plasmodium vivax and artemisinin derivatives are particularly effective against the early stages of the parasite. By combining drugs with complementary activity profiles, the treatment can effectively target multiple malaria species, providing broader coverage and improving the chances of elimination of the parasite [6, 12].

- Reduced treatment failure rates: By using drugs with different pharmacokinetic properties, the combination can provide longer-lasting effects and maintain effective drug levels in the body, improving treatment outcomes and reducing the risk of recurrent infections [6, 12].

The mechanisms of action of combination antimalarials involving quinoline drugs can vary depending on the specific drugs used. However, some common mechanisms include [6, 12]:

- Artemether-lumefantrine: This combination therapy consists of artemether, an artemisinin derivative, and lumefantrine, a quinoline derivative. It is widely used as a first-line treatment for uncomplicated malaria caused by *Plasmodium falciparum.*

- Dihydroartemisinin-piperaquine: This combination therapy involves dihydroartemisinin, an artemisinin derivative, and piperaquine, a bisquinoline derivative. It combines the rapid action of artemisinin with the longer-lasting effect of piperaquine. The combination is effective against drug-resistant strains of malaria and has been widely used as a first-line treatment.

Overall, combination antimalarials, including those involving quinoline drugs, provide increased efficacy, delayed development of drug resistance, synergistic effects, and a broader spectrum of activity. These advantages make them valuable in the treatment of uncomplicated malaria, improving patient outcomes and helping to combat the challenges posed by drug-resistant malaria strains. Despite some particular side effects limiting their use such as risk of mental confusion, vertigo, hallucination with Mefloquine; hematological disorders and liver toxicity with Amodiaquine; or even allergic manifestations such as skin erythema or photosensitization with quinine, antimalarials with a quinoline nucleus retain a place of choice in the treatment of malaria.

5. New directions in the medicinal chemistry of quinoline core antimalarials

In the area of the medicinal chemistry of quinoline core antimalarials, several advances have been made. Their objective is to improve the efficacy, safety of use and sustainably preserve these drugs from resistance. Here are some examples of notable advances:

- Development of new antimalarial derivatives: By carrying out specific structural modifications, researchers have obtained new derivatives with a quinoline nucleus with improved antimalarial activities. These modifications consisted of the introduction of atoms or functional groups on the quinoline nucleus in order to improve the antimalarial activity [19, 20].

- Combinatorial approach: Pharmacochemists are exploring how to use the chemical library and combinatorial chemistry to generate a wide range of quinoline core compounds and select those that show promising antimalarial activity. This chemoinformatics approach has led to faster discovery of new antimalarial drug candidates [4, 5, 13, 19, 20].

- Anti-resistance strategies: among the strategies for circumventing resistance to current antimalarials, some researchers propose designing compounds capable of targeting several metabolic pathways in Plasmodium [2, 20];

- Treatment personalization approach: The objective sought by adopting a personalized medicine approach is to identify the genetic markers of Plasmodium allowing the identification of the optimal treatment for each individual, taking into account the effectiveness of the drugs and the factors related to resistance [21].

- Optimization of pharmacokinetic properties: In order to ensure a sufficient concentration of the drug in infected tissues and to reduce side effects, pharmacochemists are working to improve the pharmacokinetic characteristics of antimalarials with a quinoline core, such as bioavailability, tissue distribution and half-life [13, 14].

These advances in the medicinal chemistry of quinoline antimalarials offer new perspectives for the development of more effective, safer and longer-lasting treatments for malaria. It should be noted, however, that research in this area is constantly evolving and new discoveries and innovations are likely to occur in the future.

6. Conclusion

Antimalarial drugs with quinoline patterns and analogs are a major class of antimalarial whose importance in the management of all forms of malaria has not diminished since the discovery of quinine in 1820.

The use of early quinoline core antimalarials such as chloroquine and mefloquine was associated with certain drawbacks, which motivated the development of other synthetic derivatives. Here are some of these disadvantages:

- Parasite resistance: Over time, the malaria parasite has developed resistance to certain antimalarials with a quinoline core, including chloroquine. This resistance has limited the effectiveness of these drugs in certain regions of the world, forcing the development of new therapeutic options.

- Some adverse effects specific to certain molecules limit their use in certain circumstances. Early quinoline core antimalarials showed adverse effects in some patients. For example, chloroquine can cause gastrointestinal upset, visual disturbances, and heart problems in some people. Mefloquine is also associated with side effects such as neuropsychiatric disorders, dizziness and sleep disturbances.

These disadvantages led to the research and development of new synthetic derivatives of antimalarials, such as amodiaquine, piperaquine, and pyronaridine, showing increased efficacy against malaria and better tolerance in many patients. These new therapeutic options contributed to improving the management of malaria and dealing with emerging parasitic resistance.

The quinoline nucleus remains essential for obtaining the antimalarial activities of the representatives of this class. It is necessary to respect the national protocol for the fight against malaria which proposes effective therapeutic combinations considering the characteristics of resistance specific to each population.

Author details

Deto Ursul Jean-Paul N'guessan*, Songuigama Coulibaly, Apleheni Eunice Melissa Adouko and Mahama Ouattara
University Félix Houphouët-Boigny University, Abidjan, Ivory Coast

*Address all correspondence to: jacquenguessan@gmail.com

IntechOpen

© 2023 The Author(s). Licensee IntechOpen. This chapter is distributed under the terms of the Creative Commons Attribution License (http://creativecommons.org/licenses/by/3.0), which permits unrestricted use, distribution, and reproduction in any medium, provided the original work is properly cited.

References

[1] World Malaria Report 2022. Geneva: World Health Organization; 2022. p. 372. Report No.: Licence: CC BY-NC-SA 3.0 IGO

[2] Rosenthal PJ. Antimalarial Chemotherapy: Mechanisms of Action, Resistance, and New Directions in Drug Discovery. Totowa, NY: Humana Press; 2001. p. 396. (Infectious disease)

[3] Hu YQ, Gao C, Zhang S, Xu L, Xu Z, Feng LS, et al. Quinoline hybrids and their antiplasmodial and antimalarial activities. European Journal of Medicinal Chemistry. 2017;**139**:22-47

[4] Vangapandu S, Jain M, Kaur K, Patil P, Patel SR, Jain R. Recent advances in antimalarial drug development. Medicinal Research Reviews. 2007;**27**(1):65-107

[5] Vandekerckhove S, D'hooghe M. Quinoline-based antimalarial hybrid compounds. Bioorganic & Medicinal Chemistry. 2015;**23**(16):5098-5119

[6] Scholar E. Antimalarial agents. In: Enna SJ, Bylund DB, editors. xPharm: The Comprehensive Pharmacology Reference. Cambridge, MA: S&T Books and Cell Press, Elsevier Inc; 2007. pp. 1-3. DOI: 10.1016/B978-008055232-3.61023-2

[7] Tisnerat C, Dassonville-Klimpt A, Gosselet F, Sonnet P. Antimalarial drug discovery: From quinine to the most recent promising clinical drug candidates. Current Medicinal Chemistry. 2022;**29**(19):3326-3365

[8] Graham P, editor. Antimalarial Agents: Design and Mechanism of Action. Amsterdam, Netherlands: Elsevier; 2020. p. 604

[9] Biagini GA, Bray PG, Ward SA. Mechanisms of antimalarial drug resistance. In: Mayers DL, editor. Antimicrobial Drug Resistance. Infectious Disease. New Jersey, United States: Humana Press; 2009. pp. 561-574. DOI: 10.1007/978-1-59745-180-2_40

[10] Biagini GA, Ward SA. Mechanisms of antimalarial drug resistance. In: Mayers D, Sobel J, Ouellette M, Kaye K, Marchaim D, editors. Antimicrobial Drug Resistance. Springer; 2017. pp. 629-647. DOI: 10.1007/978-3-319-46718-4_41

[11] Wicht KJ, Mok S, Fidock D. Molecular mechanisms of drug resistance in Plasmodium falciparum malaria. Annual Review of Microbiology. 2020;**74**(1):431-454

[12] Deshpande S, Kuppast B. 4-Aminoquinolines: An overview of antimalarial chemotherapy. Medicinal Chemistry. 2016;**6**:1. DOI: 10.4172/2161-0444.1000315

[13] Mishra M, Mishra VK, Kashaw V, Iyer AK, Kashaw S. Comprehensive review on various strategies for antimalarial drug discovery. European Journal of Medicinal Chemistry. 2017;**125**:1300-1320

[14] Imrat, Verma AK, Mina PR. Recent advances in antimalarial drug discovery: Challenges and opportunities. In: Tyagi RK, editor. Plasmodium Species and Drug Resistance [Internet]. London, UK: IntechOpen; 2021. Available from: https://www.intechopen.com/books/plasmodium-species-and-drug-resistance/recent-advances-in-antimalarial-drug-discovery-challenges-and-opportunities-1

[15] Foley M, Tilley L. Quinoline antimalarials: Mechanisms of action

and resistance. International Journal for Parasitology. 1997;**27**(2):231-240

[16] Bawa S, Kumar S, Drabu S, Kumar R. Structural modifications of quinoline-based antimalarial agents: Recent developments. Journal of Pharmacy & Bioallied Sciences. 2010;**2**(2):64

[17] Khan J, Kaushik M, Singh S. Molecular mechanisms of action and resistance of antimalarial drugs. In: Mandal S, Paul D, editors. Bacterial Adaptation to Co-Resistance. Berlin/Heidelberg, Germany: Springer; 2019. pp. 267-296. DOI: 10.1007/978-981-13-8503-2_14

[18] Asakawa H, Manetsch R. A comprehensive review of 4(1H)-quinolones and 4(1H)-pyridones for the development of an effective antimalarial. In: Tyagi K, editor. Plasmodium Species and Drug Resistance [Internet]. London, UK: IntechOpen; 2021. Available from: https://www.intechopen.com/books/plasmodium-species-and-drug-resistance/a-comprehensive-review-of-4-1-em-h-em-quinolones-and-4-1-em-h-em-pyridones-for-the-development-of-an

[19] Beteck R, Smit F, Haynes R, N'Da D. Recent progress in the development of anti-malarial quinolones. Malaria Journal. 2014;**13**(1):339

[20] Kucharski DJ, Jaszczak MK, Boratyński PJ. A review of modifications of quinoline antimalarials: Mefloquine and (hydroxy)chloroquine. Molecules. 2022;**27**(3):1003. DOI: 10.3390/molecules27031003

[21] Veiga MI, Peng WK. Rapid phenotyping towards personalized malaria medicine. Malaria Journal. 2020;**19**:68. DOI: 10.1186/s12936-020-3149-4